The Southern Fried Keto Foodie:
Deep Fried and Keto-fied
by
Suzanne Mosley

<u>Disclaimer:</u>
This book is for entertainment purposes only. The publisher and author of this book are not responsible for any damages arising directly or indirectly from the use of the information herein. The publisher and author disclaim any liabilities for damages caused by the use of the information found within.
No part of this book should be construed as medical advice. Consult your physician prior to making any lifestyle changes or if you have questions about whether you would benefit from eating a Keto diet.

This book is dedicated to Phillip and Tori;
my inspirations
and my greatest blessings in life.
To my dearest friends, Lee, Michelle, Kim, and Connie:
Thank you for your encouragement
and friendship.

Table of Content

Seafood Recipes:

Beef, Pork, and Venison Recipes:

Breakfast and Brunch Recipes:

Sides and Sauces:

DEEP FRIED AND KETO-FIED

Growing up in a southern home, practically all of our celebrations centered around a table full of the most amazing comfort foods and flavor packed dishes. Family reunions were an unspoken food contest and Sunday dinners were never a let down. Anytime we could find a reason to come together over food, we made sure we didn't waste the opportunity.

Throughout the years, dietary recommendations have changed. Fad diets have come and gone without any lasting results. I remember hearing some pretty crazy ideas for losing weight and thinking to myself "You can't beat genetics". I wish I would have known 13 years ago what I know now. It's not about beating genetics at all. It's about fueling each individual body with what it needs. That's when it hit me. Could I recreate my entire collection of recipes but keto style? Maybe I could.

I started with some from my grandmother's and grandfather's family recipes that were basic and simple and made little substitutions at a time. Eventually, I got bolder in my attempts. With each recipe, I became more excited that we can truly eat anything we want as long as it is prepared correctly. It was then that my keto cookbook creation was born. As my collection grew bigger and my jeans grew smaller, more and more friends have jumped on keto. This led to recipe swaps, discussions and of course, my southern food is always a big winner here in the south. This is when I decided to compile my entire collection together and put it out there for everyone to enjoy. When you get to a point where you don't see keto as 'what I can't eat' but instead see it as 'I can eat anything I want', it becomes an enjoyable way of life and the Standard American Diet seems empty.

From fried chicken to fried cabbage, country fried steak to southern salmon patties, I have altered some of the best of my recipes so that you and your family can enjoy the comfort foods that my family loves so much. Do you want to wow your family at holiday time? Try my Turducken recipe that is sure to have them asking for the recipe. Do you miss chicken pot pie? Great news! You don't have to avoid it any longer. Just cook them the keto way!

Keto has become a way of life for my family. With the ability to create virtually any food, there is hope for those like me who have fought so long to find a healthy journey that has real results. I've been a foodie all my life and now I can enjoy being a foodie without feeling guilty. From my Southern Fried Keto Foodie kitchen to yours: eat, drink, and enjoy without guilt!

The Southern Fried Keto Foodie's Guide to Tips, Tricks, and Hacks

In this cookbook, you will find that every dish can be used within the limits of the standard Ketogenic Diet of:

- Less than 20 carbs
- Moderate Protein
- Higher Fat Consumption

However, you may see that the macros fluctuate throughout the book which was by design. Clients often ask me questions like: "I have 10 grams of protein and 4 carbs left. I'm still hungry. What can I eat?" With this cookbook, you can find a recipe that will suit many needs, whether its protein you lack or you are concerned about busting your carbohydrate limit with dinner. As with any variation of a diet, there may be a few ingredients that are controversial among many Keto groups. It all boils down to personal choice. None of the ingredients I have included in my book will cause an increased insulin response.

A few things to consider:

- If you are cooking for one person, these recipes may seem like a lot of food. Use them for meal prep! This is a fantastic way to save time and money.

- Try freezing precooked chicken for an easy start to some of the recipes. It will stay fresh for 3 months.

- Oils are interchangeable! If you notice throughout my cookbook, I tend to favor bacon grease as my fat of choice. This is mainly because I was raised in a kitchen with a bacon grease jar always in reach. Choose any oil you like for these recipes. Just be sure to check for smoking point on oils that are not meant to fry over high heat.

- For those who are already "fat-adapted" and naturally moving towards One Meal A Day (OMAD), there are many recipes in here that will fit your protein and fats for the day without getting close to your carb limit.

- If you have not given intermittent fasting a try, you should look into it. My only advice is not to start intermittent fasting until you are fat adapted as you will only torture yourself. This way of life is not about restricting yourself. It's about feeling full and losing weight at the same time. Oxymoron for most, right? Not us Ketoers!

- If you use your tablet for recipes like I do, print out a kitchen measurement conversion chart and laminate it. Use adhesive spray to stick it to the inside of your tablet cover for easy access while you are cooking. You could also print out a sweetener conversion chart as well. Some Keto approved sweeteners do not convert equally so having a handy cheat sheet will be beneficial.

- Although I have nailed down the macros in these recipes to .25 of accuracy, please remember that different brands have different macros counts. For example: I have come across 3 different brands of full fat cream cheese with 3 different carb counts on them. Although the variances can be small and usually not harmful, sometimes they can cause "carb creep". This is where hidden carbs get in and push you over your carb limit unknowingly. This can cause a stall or force you out of ketosis if it is bad enough. Just keep this tidbit in mind in case you start to experience a stall. Look for carb creep first.

For the beginner:

Before getting started on Keto, here are some pointers to help you along the way.

- Keto Flu is real! Keep your electrolytes in check to minimize your symptoms and remember that it will be over in a few brief days and you will feel so much better. If you do suffer Keto Flu, remember that feeling because this is the way you will likely feel if you cheat on the plan. Introducing sugar and carbs can cause the exact same effect.

- Clear out your pantry. Take your extra food to the local community food pantry or call family members to come grocery shopping at your house. Either way, clear out everything that is not keto approved. When you are digging anywhere for sugar in that first week , thanks to the awful addiction, you will thank me later.

- Reorganize your kitchen. When you empty your pantry, do the same to your cabinets. This should leave room to move small appliances and everyday staples to the main part of your kitchen.

- Make a grocery list BEFORE you go to the store and NEVER go to the store hungry. Helpful tip: take your bullet proof coffee to the grocery store with you. The fat will keep you satisfied and you won't be tempted to become the proud owner of aisle 9.

- Special occasion coming up? Prepare ahead of time. Make sweet desserts as a meal prep to have available when everyone else is eating their inflammation extravaganza.

- There is never a stupid question when it comes to Keto. Find a good coach and a great group of supportive people and you are set up for a successful start. If you are looking to find these kind of people, feel free to join my group on Facebook:

<u>**The Southern Fried Keto Foodie**</u> and <u>**The Southern Fried Keto Foodie Support Group.**</u>

- **Don't let it overwhelm you. Start with the simplest recipes first and work towards the more difficult ones. You will learn as you go. Don't be discouraged if it takes you a little time to get it right.**

- **Most of all, take it one pound at a time. The time is going to go by anyway. Might as well make improvements as you go.**

Poultry Recipes

1 Spinach Artichoke Chicken Casserole

Ready in 1 hour

Serves 6 people

Calories: 540.5

Fat: 39

Net Carbs:3.5

Protein: 36.5

Ingredients

- **24 ounces raw chicken, sliced**
- **8 ounces frozen chopped spinach**
- **12 ounces marinaded artichoke hearts**
- **6 ounces of full fat cream cheese**
- **1/2 cup mayonnaise**
- **1/2 cup (for ingredients) / 1/2 cup (for topping) grated Parmesan**
- **1/2 cup shredded mozzarella**
- **1 tablespoon Italian Seasoning**
- **4 tablespoons bacon bits**
- **1 teaspoon garlic powder**

Kitchen Supplies

☐ large baking dish (I use glass)

☐ cutting board and sharp knife

☐ measuring cups and spoons

☐ large mixing bowl

☐ aluminum foil

Preparation

1. Preheat oven to 350 degrees. Place cream cheese out on the counter to warm up to room temperature and defrost the frozen spinach.
2. Drain your artichoke hearts. Slice Chicken breasts into 7-10 slices each and place aside.
3. In a large mixing bowl, combine all the ingredients above except for the chicken, mozzarella and 1/2 cup of Parmesan, and mix thoroughly. Add the chicken slices to the mixture and fully saturate each piece. Spread chicken and sauce in your baking pan and top with mozzarella and remaining Parmesan.
4. Cover with aluminum foil and bake for 45 minutes or until the chicken reaches an internal temperature of 165 or more. Serve hot.

Tips

To blister the cheese on top more, take the aluminum foil off the top about 35 minutes into cooking it and let it cook for 50 minutes instead. Always check the internal temperature of any dish you create before serving it. Cook times and temperatures can vary based on the type of range or oven you use.

2 Chicken Fajita Casserole

Ready in 1 hour, 15 minutes

Serves 6 people

Calories: 319

Fat: 23

Net Carbs: 4

Protein: 18

Ingredients

- **16 ounces of chicken breast, sliced**
- **2 tablespoons bacon grease**
- **4 ounces of cream cheese (softened)**
- **4 ounces of sour cream**
- **1 teaspoon of garlic powder**
- **1 teaspoon of black pepper**
- **1 teaspoon of salt**
- **1 red bell pepper, julienned**
- **1 green bell pepper, julienned**
- **1 yellow onion, julienned**
- **Salt and pepper to taste**
- **½ cup of shredded pepper jack cheese for topping and ½ cup for the mixture**

Kitchen Supplies

- ☐ cutting board and a sharp knife
- ☐ medium size mixing bowl
- ☐ large baking dish
- ☐ rubber spatula
- ☐ measuring spoons/cups

Preparation

1. **Preheat oven to 350 degrees. On a cutting board, slice your peppers and onions in a julienned fashion then slice your chicken into thin slices so that they cook quickly and evenly.**

2. Next, mix the seasonings with the cream cheese and sour cream until smooth and completely blended. Add in your peppers, onions, and 1/2 cup of pepper jack cheese and mix until it is completely incorporated.
3. Then add in the sliced chicken and saturate each piece well.
4. In a glass baking dish, add the mixture and smooth out evenly. Top with the remaining 1/2 cup of pepper jack cheese and bake for 35-40 minutes or until it is bubbly and starting to brown on top. Serve and enjoy!

Tips

Add some jalapenos or other spicy peppers for an extra kick. Serve with fresh guacamole as a topping or a side dish with celery for dipping.

3 Broiled Chicken Thighs

Ready in 1 hour, 10 minutes

Serves 10 people

Calories: 265

Fat: 19

Net Carbs: .5

Protein: 22

Ingredients

- **10 chicken thighs, bone in, skin on**
- **4 tablespoons bacon grease**
- **1/2 teaspoon rosemary**
- **1/2 teaspoon thyme**
- **1/2 teaspoon black pepper**
- **1/2 teaspoon paprika**
- **1/2 teaspoon garlic powder**
- **1/2 teaspoon cayenne pepper**
- **1 teaspoon parsley**
- **1 teaspoon oregano**
- **1 teaspoon onion powder**
- **1 teaspoon salt**

Kitchen Supplies

- ☐ Large Baking dish (I use glass)

- ☐ 2 small mixing bowls

- ☐ Tongs, measuring spoons

Preparation

1. **Preheat oven to 350 degrees. Melt bacon grease in the microwave until liquid then pour into baking dish. Blend all the spices in a bowl together and set to the side.**
2. **Take each chicken thigh and roll it around in the bacon grease in your baking pan until fully coated all the way around and place side by side in the pan for baking.**

3. Sprinkle all the seasoning evenly across all the thighs. Cover your dish with aluminum foil and bake in the oven for 45-50 minutes or until the chicken reaches an internal temperature of at least 165 degrees.
4. Take baking pan out of the oven and drain nearly all of the drippings into a bowl leaving only a tablespoon or two behind.
5. Set your oven to low broil. Bake chicken for 5-8 minutes on each side until then chicken becomes golden brown and the skin begins to crisp. Serve hot.

Tips

Save your drippings!! I keep mason jars around just for times like these. You can use your drippings for gravy or to use as stock/broth. This makes a great chicken soup base!

4 Southern Fried Chicken Tenders

Ready in 45 minutes

Serves 4 people

Calories: 335

Fat: 19

Net Carbs: 4.5

Protein: 40

Ingredients

- **16 ounces of chicken breast sliced into tenders or you can use pre-cut skinless chicken tenders**
- **4 tablespoons bacon grease**
- **1/2 teaspoon rosemary**
- **1/2 teaspoon thyme**
- **1/2 teaspoon black pepper**
- **1/2 teaspoon paprika**
- **1/2 teaspoon garlic powder**
- **1/2 teaspoon cayenne pepper**
- **1 teaspoon parsley**
- **1 teaspoon oregano**
- **1 teaspoon onion powder**
- **1 teaspoon salt**
- **¼ cup heavy whipping cream**
- **1 egg**
- **1 cup grated Parmesan cheese**
- **1 cup almond flour**

Kitchen Supplies

- ☐ Large Frying pan
- ☐ 2 small mixing bowls
- ☐ Tongs, measuring spoons

Preparation

1. **Preheat your 4 tablespoons of bacon grease in your frying pan over medium heat.**

2. Mix your egg and heavy whipping cream together to make an egg wash in one bowl and mix your seasonings, Parmesan cheese, and almond flour in another mixing bowl.
3. Put the chicken tenders in the bowl with the egg wash and saturate each of them.
4. After the egg wash, dip each tender into the dry ingredients and pat lightly on each side to adhere the coating to the chicken. Place in a single layer in the frying pan.
5. Fry each tender for 4 minutes on each side or until they reach an internal temperature of at least 165 degrees. Serve hot.

Tips

Change the seasonings to Italian and make chicken Parmesan by adding low carb marinara and mozzarella cheese over top.

5 Broccoli Cheddar Chicken

Ready in 1 hour

Serves 4 people

Calories:789.25

Fat: 34.75

Net Carbs: 6.25

Protein: 68.75

Ingredients

- **(4) 6 ounce chicken breasts**
- **1 bag of frozen broccoli**
- **½ cup of chicken broth**
- **1 cup of shredded sharp cheddar cheese**
- **¼ cup of heavy cream for sauce, ¼ cup of heavy cream for chicken breading**
- **1 teaspoon of Rotisserie chicken seasoning**
- **1/2 cup grated Parmesan cheese**
- **1 egg**
- **½ cup of almond flour**
- **1 teaspoon salt**
- **½ teaspoon of black pepper**
- **½ teaspoon of onion powder**
- **½ teaspoon of garlic powder**
- **1 tablespoon of bacon grease or butter to coat the pan**

Kitchen Supplies

- ☐ 9x9 baking pan (I use glass)
- ☐ medium sauce pan and whisk
- ☐ measuring cups and spoons
- ☐ 2 medium mixing bowls

Preparation

1. Preheat oven to 350 degrees. Melt butter or bacon grease and coat your baking pan.
2. In one mixing bowl, whisk your egg and ¼ cup of heavy whipping cream until fully combined to create an egg wash. In the other mixing bowl, combine your almond flour, Parmesan cheese, garlic powder, onion powder, salt and pepper to be used as a breading.
3. Dredge each chicken breast through the egg wash thoroughly coating on each side. Then press each side of the chicken breast into the breading combination. Pat each side to compress the breading to each chicken breast. Place each chicken breast in the baking pan not touching each other.
4. Cover with aluminum foil and bake for 45 minutes or until chicken reaches an internal temperature of 165 or more.
5. While your chicken is baking, combine the other ¼ cup of heavy cream, chicken broth, and rotisserie seasoning. Then fold in the shredded cheddar cheese. Heat over low/medium heat until melted and creamy. Set aside until chicken is done.
6. Microwave your broccoli as directed on the package. You can also choose to steam fresh broccoli as well. I use frozen because it cuts down the prep time and is more convenient for me.
7. Turn your oven to low broil or 450 degrees. Take the aluminum foil off and place the dish on the top shelf of the oven. Broil for 2-4 minutes to brown and crisp the breading.
8. Place each breast on a plate and top with broccoli and cheese sauce.

Tips

This recipe is perfect for those who do OMAD (one meal a day) plus bullet proof coffee.

6 Jalapeno Popper Chicken Casserole

Ready in 45 minutes

Serves 4 people

Calories: 500

Fat: 30.5

Net Carbs: 4.15

Protein: 43.75

Ingredients

- **16 ounces of chicken breast, diced**
- **12 strips of bacon**
- **2 fresh jalapenos**
- **4 ounces of cream cheese**
- **1 cup shredded cheddar cheese**
- **1 teaspoon of dill weed**
- **1 teaspoon of parsley**
- **1 teaspoon of onion powder**
- **1 teaspoon of garlic powder**
- **1 teaspoon of black pepper**
- **1 tablespoon of mayonnaise**

Kitchen Supplies

- ☐ cutting board and sharp knife
- ☐ large saute pan with lid
- ☐ medium baking dish
- ☐ slotted spoon, measuring cups
- ☐ medium mixing bowl

Preparation

1. **Preheat oven to 350 degrees and get out your large saute pan. Dice your chicken and place it in the saute pan and cover with a lid. Cook until the juices run clear and the chicken is done.**

2. Meanwhile, lay out your cream cheese to warm it to room temperature. Chop your bacon into crumbles and separate into two separate bowls; half for topping and half for mixing into the casserole. Also, slice your jalapenos open and clean out all of the seeds. Remember that the seeds are what make jalapenos hot so remove all the seeds if you want a milder casserole. Also remember that the longer you cook peppers, the hotter they get (because of the seeds) Feel free to leave a few seeds if you wish but it will give it a spicy bite and it can be easily overpowering if you leave too many,) Remove the stem and dice your peppers into small diced pieces.
3. In your medium mixing bowl, add your jalapenos, cream cheese, cheddar cheese, mayo, bacon crumbles, and seasonings. Mix until thoroughly blended. (Suzi Tip! I start with my wet ingredients first and then add dry ingredients to blend before adding the shredded cheddar. It seems to mix the flavors more evenly.)
4. Next, fold the cooked diced chicken into the mixture and place in a baking pan. Top with the rest of your bacon and place in the oven. Bake for 20 minutes.

Tips

As with other recipes in this book, precooking some items before combining them is key to not watering down any sauces you create. You can add more cheddar cheese to the top or use Pepper Jack for a little more spice.

7 Chicken Pizza Bake

Ready in 40 minutes

Serves 6 people

Calories: 329.75

Fat: 14.25

Net Carbs: 2.75

Protein: 43.75

Ingredients

- **24 ounces of chicken sliced**
- **30 slices of pepperoni**
- **1 cup of low carb pizza sauce**
- **1 cup of shredded mozzarella cheese**
- **2 tablespoons of grated Parmesan cheese**
- **Italian seasoning, salt, and pepper (optional)**

Kitchen Supplies

- [ ] cutting board and sharp knife
- [ ] large saute pan with lid
- [ ] medium baking dish
- [ ] slotted spoon, measuring cups/spoon

Preparation

1. **Preheat oven to 350 degrees and get out your large saute pan. Slice your chicken and place it in the saute pan and cover with a lid. Add your optional seasonings at this time. While stirring occasionally, cook until the juices run clear and the chicken is done.**
2. **Drain your chicken and lay it out in your baking pan. Pour the low carb pizza sauce over top and mix well.**
3. **Next, layer your pepperoni, mozzarella, and Parmesan over the chicken and place in the oven to bake for 20 minutes or until cheese starts to blister on top.**

Tips

Add in your favorite keto friendly pizza toppings such as mushrooms, olives, sausage, bacon, bell peppers, onions, and more. This dish is also low enough in carbs to serve with a keto bread option and seasoned olive oil for dipping.

8 Cheesy Chicken Casserole

Ready in 45 minutes

Serves 4 people

Calories: 587

Fat: 26

Net Carbs: 3.5

Protein: 66.75

Ingredients

- **24 ounces of chicken sliced**
- **1 cup of shredded cheddar cheese**
- **1 cup of chicken broth**
- **1 ounce of barbeque pork rinds**
- **1 tablespoon of butter**
- **1 bag of frozen cauliflower rice**
- **1 teaspoon of rotisserie chicken seasonings**
- **4 ounces of cream cheese**

Kitchen Supplies

- ☐ cutting board and sharp knife
- ☐ large saute pan with lid
- ☐ medium sauce pan, whisk
- ☐ 2 small mixing bowls
- ☐ medium baking dish
- ☐ slotted spoon, measuring cups/spoons

Preparation

1. **Preheat oven to 350 degrees and get out your large saute pan. Slice your chicken and place it in the saute pan and cover with a lid. You can add salt and pepper to taste at this time. While stirring occasionally, cook until the juices run clear and the chicken is done.**
2. **Meanwhile, in a medium sauce pan, combine your chicken broth, rotisserie seasoning, cream cheese and shredded cheddar cheese. Heat over low/medium and whisk frequently until your sauce is combined.**

3. Heat your cauliflower rice according to the directions on the package then spread the cauliflower rice into your baking dish.
4. Drain your chicken and lay over top of your cauliflower rice in your baking dish. Pour the cheese sauce evenly over top of the chicken and cauliflower layers.
5. In one small mixing bowl, crush up your pork rinds to bread crumb consistency. In the other mixing bowl, melt 1 tablespoon of butter. Combine the two to coat the pork rinds evenly then sprinkle them across the top of your casserole.
6. Bake your casserole uncovered for 20 minutes or until the pork rind bread crumbs start to brown and the edges are bubbly.

Tips

This is a great meal prep dish for those busy days where cooking is the least of your concerns. You can also add more shredded cheddar as a topping along with the pork rind "bread" crumbs and sprinkle with a little bit of parsley for a polished look.

9 Herb Roasted Turkey

Ready in 6 hours, 15 minutes

Serves 10 people

Calories: 449

Fat: 26.25

Net Carbs: .5

Protein: 59.75

Ingredients

- **Whole 16 pound turkey, thawed**
- **½ cup of bacon grease, room temperature**
- **1 tablespoon of rosemary**
- **1 tablespoon of thyme**
- **1 tablespoon of salt**
- **1 tablespoon of black pepper**
- **½ tablespoon of garlic powder**
- **½ tablespoon of onion powder**

Kitchen Supplies

- ☐ Turkey roasting pan
- ☐ turkey baster
- ☐ plastic wrap
- ☐ aluminum foil
- ☐ measuring cups/spoons

Preparation

1. **Preheat oven to 275 degrees. Check to make sure your turkey will fit. You may need to remove the top rack in your oven.**
2. **Add your spices to your room temperature bacon grease and combine well.**
3. **Remove the turkey neck and giblet bag from your turkey and set aside. Place your turkey in the turkey roaster. With your hands, coat your turkey with the bacon grease seasoning mixture. Use all of the mixture so that it helps season the meat.**

4. Wrap the top of your turkey roaster with plastic wrap to seal in the juices. Layer aluminum foil over the plastic wrap and seal well. Bake your turkey for approximately 6 hours. Every 2 hours, pull the turkey out and use the baster to coat the turkey in its juices then recover and put back in the oven. Turkey is done when it reaches an internal temperature of 165 degrees.

Tips

This serves well with keto "cornbread" dressing! Use your giblets to make a turkey gravy to use over both.

10 Mediterranean Stuffed Chicken

Ready in 50 minutes

Serves 4 people

Calories: 506.5

Fat: 21

Net Carbs: 5.25

Protein: 66

Ingredients

- **Four 6 ounce chicken breasts split down the middle or butterflied**
- **4 ounces of frozen chopped spinach, thawed**
- **2 ounces of sun-dried tomatoes, diced**
- **4 ounces of artichoke hearts (I use marinated in a jar)**
- **1 cup of crumbled feta cheese**
- **1 teaspoon of minced garlic**
- **1 teaspoon of salt**
- **½ teaspoon of black pepper**
- **1 teaspoon of basil**
- **1 cup of shredded mozzarella cheese**

Kitchen Supplies

- ☐ cutting board and sharp knife

- ☐ medium mixing bowl, spatula

- ☐ medium baking dish

- ☐ slotted spoon, measuring cups

Preparation

1. **Preheat oven to 350 degrees.**
2. **Butterfly or split your chicken breasts down the middle and place in your baking dish.**
3. **In your mixing bowl, combine your sun-dried tomatoes, feta cheese, salt, pepper, basil, minced garlic, artichoke hearts and spinach. Mix with your spatula until all the ingredients are fully combined with each other. This is your "stuffing".**

4. Stuff each chicken breast with the stuffing mixture and close each breast up. Any extra stuffing can be spread over top of the chicken breasts. Top with mozzarella cheese and cover with aluminum foil.
5. Bake your chicken for 40 minutes or until each piece reaches an internal temperature of 165 degrees.

Tips

Once your chicken is done, set your oven to low broil or 450 degrees. Remove the aluminum foil and place on the top rack for 2-3 minutes. This will give your entree a more finished look by blistering the cheese.

11 Down Under Chicken

Ready in 50 minutes

Serves 4 people

Calories: 698

Fat: 39.75

Net Carbs: 1.5

Protein: 65.5

Ingredients

- **Four 6 ounce chicken breasts, butterflied**
- **8 strips of bacon**
- **4 tablespoons of my honey mustard recipe (It's in this book!)**
- **4 ounces of fresh mushroom slices**
- **2 tablespoons of butter**
- **1 cup of shredded Monterey Jack cheese**

Kitchen Supplies

- ☐ cutting board and sharp knife
- ☐ medium saute pan with lid
- ☐ medium baking dish
- ☐ measuring cups

Preparation

1. **Preheat oven to 350 degrees. Butterfly your chicken breasts and lay them flat in your baking dish. Cover with aluminum foil and cook for 35 minutes.**
2. **In your saute pan, melt 1 tablespoon of butter. Next, add your mushrooms and saute until al dente. Set aside until the chicken comes out at the 35 minute mark.**
3. **Scoop one ounce of mushrooms on top of each chicken breast. Then, pour 1 tablespoon of honey mustard over the mushrooms as evenly as possible. Finish by topping each breast with a ¼ cup of shredded monterey jack cheese.**
4. **Bake an additional 15-20 minutes until the cheese is bubbly and the internal temperature reaches 165 degrees.**

Tips

Swap the honey mustard with keto friendly barbeque sauce and replace the mushrooms with sauteed onions for a western flare.

12 Chicken Waffles

Ready in 40 minutes

Serves 4 people

Calories: 214

Fat: 19

Net Carbs: 2.75

Protein: 10

Ingredients

- **2/3 cup of coconut flour**
- **12 large eggs**
- **1 teaspoon of vanilla extract**
- **3 tablespoons of erythritol**
- **8 tablespoons of melted butter**
- **1 tsp of salt**
- **1 teaspoon of baking powder**

Kitchen Supplies

☐ small waffle maker

☐ blender

☐ Rubber spatula

☐ measuring spoons/cup

Preparation

1. **Preheat your small waffle maker.**
2. **In your blender, add all 12 of your eggs, and your melted butter. Blend well.**
3. **Next, add in your vanilla extract, erythritol, salt, baking powder and coconut flour. Blend until fully incorporated.**
4. **Pour about ½ cup of batter onto your small waffle maker. If you are using a larger one, double the portion to 1 cup of batter. Just remember to double count your macros.**
5. **Cook waffles until they are golden brown. Serve hot.**

Tips

I call these chicken waffles because they are perfect to pair with my southern fried chicken tenders for chicken and waffles night! Smother them in butter and sugar free maple syrup. These waffles are so tasty that if you never told your family they are keto, they would never know.

13 Chicken Pot Pie

Ready in 1 hour

Serves 6 people

Calories: 572

Fat: 38.25

Net Carbs: 9.5

Protein: 45

Ingredients

Filling:

- **16 ounces of diced chicken breast**
- **4 tablespoons bacon grease**
- **2 bunches of radishes (about 20 each)**
- **1 bag frozen Italian cut green beans**
- **1/2 teaspoon onion powder**
- **1 teaspoon salt**
- **1 teaspoon black pepper**
- **6 pieces of bacon crumbled**
- **Sauce:**
- **1 teaspoon McCormick Rotisserie Chicken seasonings**
- **3 tablespoons sour cream**
- **1 1/3 cups chicken broth**
- **1/2 cup shredded cheddar cheese**
- **2 tablespoons cream cheese**
- **1 teaspoon xantham gum**
  Crust:
- **1/2 teaspoon McCormick Rotisserie Chicken seasonings**
- **1/2 cup shredded cheddar cheese**
- **2 tablespoons cream cheese**
- **1 cup almond flour**
- **1 egg**
- **1 1/2 cups shredded mozzarella cheese**

Kitchen Supplies

- ☐ Large Saute Pan with lid

- ☐ medium baking dish (I use glass)

- ☐ Measuring spoons/cups

- ☐ Mixing bowl

- ☐ cutting board and sharp knife

- ☐ slotted spoon

- ☐ small sauce pot

- ☐ rubber spatula

Preparation

1. **Preheat oven to 350 degrees. You need to already have your bacon cooked and ready to crumble. An easy way to do this is to bake it in the oven on parchment paper at 325 degrees until crispy. Hand crumble the bacon and set aside. Take one tablespoon of bacon grease and coat the inside of your baking dish.**
2. **Next, melt the other 3 tablespoons of bacon grease in a large saute pan. Dice 16 ounces of chicken breast into 1/2 inch pieces and place in the saute pan with the bacon grease. Add salt and pepper. Cook until juices run clear and chicken is done. Use your slotted spoon to remove the cooked chicken and set aside.**
3. **While the chicken is cooking, cut the ends off the radishes and dice them into quarters unless they are smaller then you need to cut them in half. You do not have to defrost the green beans. You can add them frozen in the next step.**
4. **In the juices remaining in the saute pan, add your radishes and green beans. Add in the onion powder and let simmer until radishes are soft and green beans are cooked. Drain all of this and set aside with your chicken and bacon.**
5. **In another small sauce pot, add your chicken stock, cream cheese, sour cream, cheddar cheese, and chicken seasoning. Heat over low to medium heat stirring every couple minutes with a rubber spatula to keep the cheese sauce from sticking and scorching. Heat until everything is fully melted and blended.**
6. **Mix the chicken, bacon, and veggies in a bowl together and add cheese sauce. Use your spatula to fold the sauce into the ingredients so that you don't crush the radishes. Add all of this to the baking pan.**
7. **In another mixing bowl, add the cream cheese for the crust and mozzarella cheese. Place the bowl in the microwave for a minute. The mozzarella should be melted and the cream cheese should be easy to incorporate into it.**

8. Next, add the egg, seasoning, and almond flour. Blend and knead these five ingredients until they are fully combined and have a dough texture. Add the cheddar cheese and continue to fully incorporate all ingredients.

9. Lay a piece of parchment paper over your cutting board. (You can also use plastic wrap for this) Lay the dough on the parchment paper and roll out until it is the size of your baking dish. Lay the dough/parchment paper on a baking sheet and bake for 8 minutes or until the edges start to turn brown. Pick up the crust and lay browned side down on top of the casserole. Tuck the ends of the crust into the sides of the dish so that they don't burn before your pot pie is finished baking.

10. Place pot pie in the oven for 20 minutes or until the crust starts to brown and look crisp. Remove from the oven and let it sit for about 10 minutes then serve hot.

Tips

The reason I precook my ingredients before assembling this recipe is because chicken holds water and so do green beans and radishes. If yo u allow those juices to combine with the sauce , you will end up with a watery sauce when you serve it. In order to keep the consistency of the sauce with typical pot pie sauce, you cannot add any extra liquid to the filling.

14 Smothered Chicken

Ready in 40 minutes

Serves 4 people

Calories: 482.5

Fat: 22

Net Carbs: 7.5

Protein: 60

Ingredients

- **Four 6 ounce chicken breasts**
- **2 cups sliced mushrooms**
- **1 cup of beef broth**
- **2 tablespoons of bacon grease**
- **salt and pepper to taste**
- **1 teaspoon of minced garlic**
- **1 cup of julienned yellow onion**
- **½ teaspoon of rosemary**
- **½ teaspoon of thyme**
- **a pinch of xantham gum**
- **4 slices of white cheddar cheese**

Kitchen Supplies

- cutting board and sharp knife
- medium baking dish (I use glass)
- large iron skillet, tongs
- slotted spoon, whisk, measuring cups and spoons

Preparation

1. **Preheat oven to 400 degrees. Slice your mushrooms and julienne cut your onions.**
2. **In your large iron skillet, melt 2 tablespoons of bacon grease. Add your chicken breasts and cover to cook for 25 minutes over medium heat. Flip at least once to sear the outside. When the chicken reaches an internal**

temperature of 165 degrees, put chicken aside and leave the chicken drippings in the skillet.

3. In the same large skillet, add your mushrooms and onions. Cover and cook them for 8-10 minutes over medium heat until they are soft. Use your slotted spoon to remove the mushrooms and onions and set aside.

4. Add your 1 cup of beef broth, whisk into the drippings, and bring to a simmer. Add your minced garlic, rosemary, thyme, salt, and pepper. Continue whisking until it reaches a high simmer. Lower the heat to low.medium and add a pinch of xantham gum at a time and give it a couple minutes in between to thicken before adding the next. You are looking only for it to lightly coat the spoon.

5. In your baking dish, line your four chicken breasts up and evenly top with mushrooms and onions. Pour half the sauce over the mushrooms and onions. Next, lay a slice of white cheddar cheese over each chicken breast. Drizzle the remaining sauce over top of the cheese.

6. Place your baking dish on the top rack of the oven and bake for 15-20 minutes or until the cheese starts to blister.

Tips

Bacon makes a great addition to personalize this dish.

15 Chicken Broccoli Alfredo Casserole

Ready in 45 minutes

Serves 6 people

Calories: 447

Fat: 37

Net Carbs: 3.7

Protein: 31.5

Ingredients

- **16 ounces of chicken breast, diced**
- **1 bag frozen broccoli**
- **6 tablespoons butter**
- **1 cup heavy cream**
- **1 cup grated Parmesan cheese**
- **1/2 teaspoon of salt**
- **1/2 teaspoon black pepper**
- **1 clove of garlic grated or minced**
- **1/2 cup of shredded mozzarella**

Kitchen Supplies

- ☐ cutting board and sharp knife
- ☐ large saute pan with lid
- ☐ medium baking dish
- ☐ slotted spoon, measuring cups
- ☐ small sauce pan

Preparation

1. **Preheat oven to 350 degrees and get out your large saute pan. Dice your chicken and place it in the saute pan and cover with a lid. Cook until the juices run clear and the chicken is done.**
2. **Meanwhile, microwave your broccoli and rough cut it into bite sized pieces.**

3. To make the sauce, add the 6 tablespoons of butter to the sauce pan and let melt over low/med heat. When the butter is melted, add salt, pepper, and heavy cream. As the heavy cream heats and you start to see small bubbles, add the Parmesan cheese and stir constantly until sauce is well incorporated and the Parmesan has melted. This is a traditional Alfredo sauce and therefore is not as thick as most people believe Alfredo sauce should be. If you want a thicker sauce, add a teaspoon of xantham gum but add it in by sprinkling it so that it doesn't clump in the sauce.
4. In a glass baking pan, add the cooked chicken and broccoli. Pour your Alfredo sauce evenly over top then sprinkle the mozzarella cheese over top. Cook for 20 minutes or until cheese starts to brown or blister. Serve hot.

Tips

As with other recipes in this book, precooking some items before combining them is key to not watering down any sauces you create.

16 Cajun Chicken Alfredo

Ready in 45 minutes

Serves 6 people

Calories: 532

Fat: 34

Net Carbs: 2

Protein: 48.25

Ingredients

- **24 ounces of sliced chicken breast**
- **1 cup of shredded Parmesan cheese**
- **1 tablespoon of Cajun seasonings**
- **1 cup of heavy whipping cream**
- **2 tablespoons of butter**
- **1 ½ cups of shredded monterey jack cheese**
- **A pinch of xantham gum**
- **1 tablespoon of bacon grease**
- **salt to taste**

Kitchen Supplies

- ☐ Large iron skillet with lid
- ☐ cutting board and sharp knife
- ☐ slotted spoon, whisk, measuring cups and spoons

Preparation

1. **Preheat your oven to 350 degrees. Slice your chicken into roughly 1/8 inch thick. Place the sliced chicken into the skillet with a tablespoon of bacon grease. Cook chicken over medium heat until the juices run clear and all the pink is gone. Use your slotted spoon and remove the chicken to set aside.**
2. **Turn down the heat under the skillet to low/medium heat and add the 2 tablespoons of butter. Whisk consistently until the butter melts completely into the chicken drippings. Add your Cajun seasoning, salt, and heavy whipping cream and blend well with your whisk. Lastly, add in 1 cup of shredded Parmesan and whisk until your Alfredo sauce is**

smooth. If your sauce seems to thin, add xantham gum a pinch at a time until you get your preferred consistency.

3. **Toss your chicken back into the skillet with your Alfredo sauce and stir together.**

4. **Without removing from the skillet, evenly top the entree with monterey jack cheese and put the skillet in the oven for 15-17 minutes or until the cheese blisters and the edges are bubbly.**

Tips

Serve with steamed broccoli or over spaghetti squash. Spice it up by adding andouille sausage or chorizo.

17 Chicken and Asparagus Bake

Ready in 1 hour

Serves 4 people

Calories: 562

Fat: 27.5

Net Carbs: 5.5

Protein: 68.75

Ingredients

- 24 ounces of chicken, sliced
- 1 pound of asparagus, ends trimmed, cut into 2 inch pieces
- 3 tablespoons of lemon juice
- 6 slices of Havarti cheese
- 2 tablespoons of liquid aminos
- ½ cup of chicken broth
- 2 teaspoons of minced garlic
- 2 tablespoons of bacon grease
- ¼ cup of bacon bits
- ½ teaspoon of xantham gum
- 1 tablespoon of ginger
- Salt and pepper (to taste)

Kitchen Supplies

- cutting board and a sharp knife
- large saute pan with lid
- large baking dish
- 2 bowls
- measuring spoons/cups, large slotted spoon

Preparation

1. Preheat oven to 350 degrees. On a cutting board, trim your asparagus ends. You want to trim away the purple at the bottom as the ends tend to be grain-y. Cut your asparagus into 2 inch pieces and lay them aside. Next, slice your chicken breasts into ¼ inch slices

2. Heat your 2 tablespoons of bacon grease over medium heat in your saute pan and add chicken. Cover and let cook, stirring occasionally, until the juices run clear and it temps at 165 degrees or higher. Use a slotted spoon to move the chicken to another bowl. Add your asparagus minced garlic, salt and pepper. Stir and cover with the lid. Cook for 8 minutes over medium heat. Remove the lid and add in your ginger, chicken broth/xantham gum/liquid aminos sauce, and lemon juice. Heat to a simmer and add your chicken back in and mix together.

3. Pour the contents of your saute pan into a large baking dish. Cover the entree with your Havarti cheese slices and bacon bits, and place the dish in the oven for 20 minutes or until cheese is melted and the dish is bubbly around the sides. Serve hot.

Tips

This goes great with cauliflower rice as a stir fry style entree.

18 Lemon and Thyme Roasted Chicken

Ready in 1 hour

Serves 6 people

Calories: 336

Fat: 20.75

Net Carbs: 2

Protein: 32.25

Ingredients

- **6 chicken thighs, skin on**
- **1 lemon cut into 6 round thin slices**
- **1 tablespoon of fresh thyme**
- **¼ cup of lemon juice**
- **1 teaspoon of xantham gum**
- **1 teaspoon of onion powder**
- **2 teaspoons of minced garlic**
- **2 teaspoons of erythritol**
- **Salt and pepper (to taste)**
- **¼ cup of heavy cream**
- **2 tablespoons of butter**
- **2 tablespoons of bacon grease**

Kitchen Supplies

- ☐ cutting board and a sharp knife
- ☐ medium sauce pan
- ☐ small bowl, spoon
- ☐ baking sheet with rim
- ☐ whisk, measuring spoons/cups

Preparation

1. Preheat oven to 350 degrees. Coat each chicken thigh with bacon grease. Be sure to saturate the skin really well and place the chicken on your baking sheet skin side up.
2. In a small bowl, mix your thyme, onion powder, salt and pepper. Sprinkle only half of this across your chicken thighs.
3. Bake your chicken thighs for 30 minutes or until they reach an internal temperature of 165 degrees.
4. Meanwhile, in your sauce pan, add your lemon juice over medium heat and reduce it by half. Add your butter and erythritol over low heat whisking frequently so you don't break the butter. Then add your heavy whipping cream and whisk to incorporate. Heat until it simmers. Add in your xantham gum and whisk continuously until it is fully incorporated and the sauce starts to thicken enough to coat a spoon lightly. Remove from heat and set aside until the chicken is done.
5. Place the chicken on a plate and drizzle the lemon cream sauce over top. Serve hot.

Tips

Add radishes to the pan with the chicken as it cook. They make a great replacements for potatoes.

19 Skillet Chicken with Paprika Cream Sauce

Ready in 45 minutes

Serves 4 people

Calories: 703.5

Fat: 43

Net Carbs: 3

Protein: 69

Ingredients

- **24 ounces of sliced raw chicken**
- **2 tablespoons Bacon Grease**
- **3/4 cup heavy whipping cream**
- **1 1/2 tablespoons paprika**
- **1 teaspoon each of salt and pepper**
- **1 teaspoon garlic powder**
- **1.2 cup of shredded cheddar cheese**
- **1 cup grated Parmesan cheese**
- **1 cup chicken broth**

Kitchen Supplies

- Large Saute pan
- Tongs, Large spoon
- cutting board and sharp knife
- measuring spoons/cups

Preparation

1. **In a large saute pan, melt bacon grease over low heat. While the bacon grease is getting hot, slice chicken into approximately 7-10 pieces about a 1/4 inch thick.**

2. Increase the heat to medium and add chicken slices in a single layer. Cook thoroughly until juices run clear and each side is browned slightly. Remove the chicken from the pan and place aside. Do not drain the pan.
3. Turn the heat back down to medium/low and add chicken broth, heavy whipping cream, seasonings, and cheeses, then mix well. Continue to stir until the sauce is well blended and smooth.
4. Add the chicken to the sauce and saturate each piece. Shingle chicken slices on a plate and top with additional sauce. Serve hot.

Tips

For an added flare, sprinkle your favorite seasoning, such as cilantro or parsley, over top as a garnish.

20 Chicken Cordon Blue Bake

Ready in 45 minutes

Serves 4 people

Calories: 694

Fat: 41-5

Net Carbs: 5

Protein: 73.75

Ingredients

- **24 ounces of sliced chicken breast raw**
- **½ pound of black forest ham, diced or shredded**
- **2 tablespoons of bacon grease**
- **6 slices of Swiss cheese**
- **½ cup of my honey mustard (see the recipe in this book)**

Kitchen Supplies

- cutting board and a sharp knife
- large baking dish
- aluminum foil
- measuring spoon/cup

Preparation

1. **Preheat oven to 350 degrees. On a cutting board, slice your chicken into thin pieces.**
2. **Take half of your black forest ham and scatter it in the bottom of the baking dish. Layer the chicken over the ham. Next, pour the honey mustard sauce evenly over the dish. Layer the rest of the black forest ham and then top it with slices of cream cheese.**
3. **Cover the dish with aluminum foil and bake for 35 minutes. Remove the aluminum foil and place the dish on the top rack. Bake for 10 more minutes until the dish is bubbly and the cheese starts to blister on top. Serve hot.**

Tips
Save time and buy a rotisserie chicken or already precooked chicken to start.

21 Garlic Parmesan Chicken

Ready in 40 minutes

Serves 4 people

Calories: 585

Fat: 32.5

Net Carbs: .25

Protein: 54.5

Ingredients

- **Four 6 ounce chicken breasts**
- **1 teaspoon of garlic powder**
- **2 tablespoons of grated Parmesan cheese**
- **Salt and pepper (to taste)**
- **2 tablespoons of bacon bits**
- **½ cup of mayonnaise**

Kitchen Supplies

- ☐ large baking dish
- ☐ aluminum foil
- ☐ small bowl, standard spoon
- ☐ measuring spoons/cups

Preparation

1. **Preheat oven to 350 degrees. Melt your bacon grease in the microwave. Pour the melted bacon grease in the bottom of your baking dish and lay your four chicken breasts spaced evenly apart.**
2. **In a small bowl, mix your mayonnaise, Parmesan cheese, garlic, salt, and pepper. Mix well. Then evenly coat the top of each chicken breast.**
3.
4. **Cover your dish with aluminum foil and bake for 35 minutes or until the juices run clear and the internal temperature reaches a minimum of 165 degrees. Sprinkle your bacon bits as a garnish. Serve hot.**

Tips
Add mozzarella on top or just add more Parmesan for a richer sauce.

22 Turducken

Ready in 9 hours

Serves 25 people

Calories: 535.75

Fat: 15.75

Net Carbs: .75

Protein: 62.5

Ingredients

- **18 pound whole turkey**
- **5 pound whole chicken**
- **3 pound whole duck**
- **½ cup of bacon grease**
- **1 tablespoon of rosemary**
- **1 tablespoon of garlic powder**
- **1 tablespoon of paprika**
- **1 tablespoon of onion powder**
- **1 tablespoon of salt**
- **2 tablespoons of brown sugar alternative (sugar free)**
- **2 tablespoons of crushed red pepper flakes**
- **1 time batch of my Keto Dressing (included in this cookbook)**

Kitchen Supplies

- ☐ large roasting pan
- ☐ small bowl, spoon
- ☐ Rubber spatula, kitchen shears, slotted spoon
- ☐ plastic wrap, aluminum foil
- ☐ measuring spoons/cups

Preparation

1. Preheat oven to 300 degrees. Remove the giblets from your foul and set them aside for later. Remove the neck and discard or save to make broth from.
2. Make a one time batch of my keto dressing but don't bake it. Mix your rosemary, garlic powder, paprika, onion powder, crushed red pepper flakes,

salt, and brown sugar alternative in a bowl. Take your bacon grease and coat the outside of all three foul. In order to make sure your foul will fit, you may have to use kitchen sheers to cut down the back side of the ribs so each foul will fit inside the other. Coat all three of your foul with the seasoning blend.

3. Take your chicken and stuff it inside your turkey. Take your dressing and stuff it between the skins of the chicken and the turkey. Pack it in all the way around. Next, stuff your duck into your chicken. Now, pack dressing between the chicken and the duck. You should have just enough dressing left to stuff the inside of the duck.

4. Cover your roasting pan with plastic wrap. Next, cover the plastic wrap with aluminum foil.

5. Bake in the oven for 8 hours or until the duck reaches an internal temperature of 165 degrees.

6. Let your dish cool before preparing it. As you carve each bird, shred it into bite sized pieces. Scoop out the dressing into another bowl with a slotted spoon. Place your meat in another bowl. If you use an oven safe dish to put these in, you can set your oven to 200 degrees and place them in there to keep them warm while you carve the next foul. Continue to repeat the process until most of the dressing is out of the pan and you have pulled all the meat from the bones.

7. One a decorative platter, Mix the meats together evenly and pile them across the tray. Use the dressing to pour it down the center of the meat on the tray in a line. Garnish with parsley for a finished look.

Tips

Take your giblets and make my giblet gravy! This recipe makes for a fantastic holiday meal to wow your family. They will never believe it doesn't even have an entire carb per serving!

23 White Cheddar Chicken Casserole

Ready in 1 hour, 15 minutes

Serves 6 people

Calories: 448.5

Fat: 18.75

Net Carbs: 5

Protein: 60.5

Ingredients

- **24 ounces of chicken breast, diced or shredded**
- **1 tablespoon of bacon grease**
- **¼ cup of heavy whipping cream**
- **1 teaspoon of minced garlic**
- **2 tablespoons of butter**
- **1 medium spaghetti squash**
- **½ cup of shredded white cheddar cheese**
- **1 package of white cheddar spreadable cheese wedges**
- **2 ounces of cream cheese**
- **Salt and pepper (to taste)**

Kitchen Supplies

- ☐ cutting board and a sharp knife

- ☐ medium sauce pan

- ☐ large saute pan with lid

- ☐ large baking sheet

- ☐ Rubber spatula

- ☐ measuring spoons/cups

Preparation

1. **Preheat your oven to 350 degrees. Cut your spaghetti squash in half and scoop out the seeds much like a pumpkin. Melt one tablespoon of butter and**

coat the insides of each half of the spaghetti squash and place them skin up on a baking sheet. Bake for 45 minutes or until you can squeeze the squash. It will be soft and mushy from the outside shell.

2. Dice your chicken and add it to your saute pan with your bacon grease. Heat over medium with the lid on, stirring occasionally until the juices run clear and your chicken temps out at 165 degrees.

3. Meanwhile, add your remaining tablespoon of butter to a medium sauce pan and turn the heat on low. Melt the butter slowly to prevent breaking. Once the butter melts, add your minced garlic, salt and pepper, cream cheese, and cheese wedges. Turn the heat to low/medium and stir frequently to prevent sticking.

4. Pull your spaghetti squash out of the oven and them over. Let them cool a bit and then take a fork and scrape the insides of the spaghetti squash out into your baking dish. The only thing you should discard is the shell. Spread your spaghetti squash evenly in the bottom of the dish.

5. Next, drain your chicken and layer it evenly over the spaghetti squash then pour the white cheddar sauce over top. Top with shredded white cheddar and place in the oven to bake for 20 minutes or until the white cheddar blisters on top and the casserole is bubbly around the sides. Serve hot.

Tips

Broccoli, Bacon, Sliced Bratwurst or diced pepperoni make great additions. You can also replace the spaghetti squash with cauliflower rice if you want to cut back on some prep time.

24 Phillip's Feel Better Chicken Soup

Ready in 1 hour, 30 minutes

Serves 10 people

Calories: 441

Fat: 9

Net Carbs: 4.75

Protein: 69.75

Ingredients

- 5 pounds of chicken breast, diced
- 1 pound of radishes, trimmed and halved
- 96 ounces of chicken broth
- 10 stalks of celery, diced
- 1 bunch of cilantro chopped fine
- 1 cup of yellow onion diced fine
- 2 jalapenos, diced fine, de-seeded
- 1 red bell pepper, diced fine
- Salt and pepper (to taste)
- 2 tablespoons of lemon juice
- 1 tablespoon of minced garlic
- 1 teaspoon of paprika

Kitchen Supplies

- ☐ cutting board and a sharp knife

- ☐ large stock pot with a lid

- ☐ measuring spoons/cups, soup ladle

Preparation

1. Dice your chicken and add it along with the chicken broth to the stock pot. Set your heat to high and cover the pot with a lid.
2. As the chicken boils, cut up your produce and put to the side.
3. Add your lemon juice, paprika, minced garlic, salt and pepper to your stock pot and stir occasionally. Boil your soup, covered, over high heat for 25

minutes. **Then add your produce to the stock pot and turn the heat down to medium. Let your soup simmer for 30-40 minutes.**

Tips

My husband is famous for his Feel Better Chicken Soup so I thought it was only right of me to name it after him. This soup is packed with so many antioxidants and vitamins that it is sure to hit the spot on those days when you feel under the weather.

25 Caesar Chicken Salad

Ready in 45 minutes

Serves 4 people

Calories: 524.5

Fat: 41.25

Net Carbs: 3

Protein: 39.5

Ingredients

- **1 pound of chicken breast, diced**
- **5 stalks of fresh celery, chopped**
- **½ cup of chopped pecans**
- **½ cup of shredded Parmesan cheese**
- **½ cup of keto-friendly Caesar dressing**
- **Salt and pepper (to taste)**

Kitchen Supplies

- [ ] cutting board and a sharp knife
- [ ] medium saute pan with a lid
- [ ] medium mixing bowl
- [ ] Rubber spatula
- [ ] measuring cups

Preparation

1. **On your cutting board, chop your celery, then dice up your chicken. Set your celery to the side and put your diced chicken, salt, and pepper in the saute pan and cover with a lid. Heat over medium heat for 20 minutes stirring occasionally. The chicken should reach an internal temperature of 165 degrees. Use a slotted spoon and remove the chicken from the saute pan and place in a medium mixing bowl. Place the bowl in the freezer to "flash cool" your chicken. You want your chicken to be below 40 degrees.**
2. **Once your chicken reaches the proper cooled stage, toss in the remaining ingredients and mix well. Cover and refrigerate.**

Tips
Add some bacon bits or red bell peppers for a little extra flavor.

Seafood Recipes

26 Southern Salmon Patties with Sriracha Cream Sauce

Ready in 30 minutes

Serves 6 people

Calories: 287/86

Fat: 19/9

Net Carbs: 3/1

Protein: 20/.25

Ingredients

Salmon Patties:

- **(1) 14.75 ounce can pink salmon, de-boned**
- **3 tablespoons Bacon Grease**
- **1 cup almond flour**
- **1/4 cup grated Parmesan**
- **1 teaspoon onion powder**
- **1/2 teaspoon garlic powder**
- **Salt and Pepper to taste**
- **2 eggs**

Sriracha Cream Sauce:

- **1/4 cup mayonnaise**
- **2 tablespoons heavy whipping cream**
- **1 1/2 tablespoons sriracha sauce**
- **1/2 teaspoon garlic powder**

Kitchen Supplies

- ☐ Large Cast Iron Skillet

- ☐ spatula for flipping patties

- ☐ large spoon, measuring spoons/cups

- ☐ medium mixing bowl, 2 small mixing bowls

Preparation

1. In a large cast iron skillet, preheat bacon grease on medium heat.
2. Open salmon, debone completely, and place in medium sized mixing bowl.
3. Next beat the eggs and heavy cream in a small mixing bowl then add to the salmon.
4. Add almond flour, Parmesan cheese, and spices; mix thoroughly and patty into six portions.
5. Add all six patties to the heated bacon grease and fry on each side for about 5 minutes or until golden brown.
6. While the salmon patties are frying, combine all the ingredients for the sauce in a small mixing bowl until smooth. Drizzle cold over top of the hot salmon patties as a finishing sauce.

Tips

For a more coastal flavor, add a teaspoon of dried cilantro and a teaspoon of lemon juice to the salmon patty mixture before frying.

27 Shrimp Scampi

Ready in 1 hour

Serves 4 people

Calories: 430

Fat: 42

Net Carbs: 11

Protein: 21.25

Ingredients

- **1 pound of raw jumbo shrimp, peeled/deveined**
- **10 tablespoons of butter**
- **1 ½ cups of Sauvignon Blanc**
- **1 teaspoon of Italian seasoning**
- **3 teaspoons of minced garlic**
- **2 tablespoons of lemon juice**
- **1 teaspoon of salt**

Kitchen Supplies

- ☐ large saute pan
- ☐ whisk, large spoon
- ☐ medium bowl
- ☐ measuring spoons

Preparation

1. **Put your white wine and lemon juice in your saute pan and reduce over medium heat. The amount of liquid should reduce by half. Turn the heat down to low/medium and add 8 tablespoons of butter. Whisk slowly but frequently to keep the butter from breaking as you melt it into your sauce. Add your minced garlic, Italian seasoning, and salt and mix them in.**
2. **Pour your sauce into a separate bowl and set aside. Turn the heat back up to medium and add the other two tablespoons of butter to the pan. Once melted, add your shrimp and cook thoroughly.**
3. **Once your shrimp are done, pour your sauce back into the saute pan. Serve hot.**

Tips

A traditional scampi does not include Parmesan over top like you get at so many restaurants. Sprinkle Parmesan over your dish to give it more of a restaurant style flavor.

28 Crab Cakes with Cajun Cream Sauce

Ready in 30 minutes

Serves 4 people

Calories: 386.5

Fat: 102.75

Net Carbs: 3

Protein: 35

Ingredients

- **1 pound of lump crab meat**
- **1 tablespoon of bacon grease**
- **½ cup of grated Parmesan cheese**
- **Salt and pepper (to taste)**
- **1 egg**
- **½ teaspoon of lemon juice**
- **1 tablespoon of cilantro**
- **1 teaspoon of paprika**
- **¼ cup of heavy whipping cream**
- **2 ounces of cream cheese**
- **1 tablespoon of Cajun seasoning**
- **¼ cup of chicken broth**
- **½ teaspoon of garlic powder**

Kitchen Supplies

- ☐ medium size mixing bowl
- ☐ medium sauce pan
- ☐ large iron skillet
- ☐ whisk, spatula, measuring spoons/cups

Preparation

1. **Preheat your bacon grease in your skillet.**

2. In your mixing bowl, combine your lump crab meat, cilantro, paprika, lemon juice, salt and pepper to taste, almond flour, garlic powder, Parmesan cheese, and egg until you can form nice thick patties with well incorporated ingredients.
3. Place your crab cakes in the hot bacon grease and fry on each side for approximately 5-7 minutes. You want the internal temperature to reach 165 degrees.
4. Meanwhile, in your sauce pan, combine the chicken broth, cream cheese, heavy cream, and Cajun seasoning. Whisk frequently over low/medium heat until smooth and hot.
5. Place your crab cake on a plate and drizzle your Cajun cream sauce over top.

Tips

I love adding Serrano or jalapenos to make them spicy. You can also add a tablespoon of horseradish if you like an extra kick.

29 Parmesan Crusted Salmon

Ready in 45 minutes

Serves 4 people

Calories: 647

Fat: 46

Net Carbs: .75

Protein: 54.5

Ingredients

- **Four 8 ounce salmon fillets, skin off**
- **2 tablespoons of grated Parmesan**
- **½ ounce of pork rinds**
- **2 teaspoons of dill weed**
- **1 tablespoon of butter**
- **4 tablespoons of mayonnaise**
- **1 tablespoon of creamy horseradish**
- **1 teaspoon of minced garlic**
- **Salt and pepper (to taste)**

Kitchen Supplies

- ☐ 3 small mixing bowl
- ☐ large baking dish
- ☐ measuring spoons, spoon

Preparation

1. **Preheat oven to 350 degrees. Melt your butter in the microwave. Take ½ tablespoon of butter and coat your dish. Lay your salmon in the dish evenly spaced apart.**
2. **In your small mixing bowl, mix your mayonnaise, creamy horseradish, minced garlic, dill weed, salt, and pepper. Mix well.**
3. **Coat each salmon fillet with your mayonnaise mixture.**
4. **Crush your pork rinds to bread crumb size in a small mixing bowl. Take the other ½ tablespoon of butter and mix with the pork rinds until they are all lightly coated. Toss in your grated Parmesan cheese and mix well.**
5. **Sprinkle your bread crumb mixture evenly over each of the salmon fillets.**

6. Bake for 20-25 minutes or until the pork rinds are browning and the juices are bubbly. Serve hot.

Tips

I have taken the left overs from this dish and mashed them into a dip and added a little sour cream creating a salmon spread for keto bagels and crackers.

30 Southern Fried Catfish

Ready in 40 minutes

Serves 8 people

Calories: 573.5

Fat: 32.5

Net Carbs: 3

Protein: 65

Ingredients

- 8 medium sized boneless catfish fillets
- ½ cup of almond flour
- 1 cup of grated Parmesan cheese
- ½ cup of coconut flour
- ¼ cup of heavy whipping cream
- 1 ogg
- 1 tablespoon of Cajun seasonings
- 6 tablespoons of bacon grease or olive oil

Kitchen Supplies

- ☐ Large saute pan
- ☐ tongs, fork, measuring cups, and spoons
- ☐ 2 small mixing bowls
- ☐ Large plate, paper towels

Preparation

1. In a large saute pan, heat your bacon grease or olive oil over low/medium heat to a temperature of at least 350 degrees.
2. In one of your small mixing bowls, combine your egg and heavy whipping cream then whip with a fork until well blended. This will be your egg wash
3. In the other small mixing bowl, add your Parmesan, almond flour, coconut flour, and Cajun seasoning. Mix all the dry ingredients well. This will be your "breading".
4. Handling gently, coat each fillet in the egg wash and then the breading. Place each fillet in the bacon grease to cook for 8 minutes on each side or until

dark golden brown and the internal temperature reaches 165 degrees. Be careful not to flip or turn your fillets too often as the breading will fall off.

5. When the fillets are done, place them on a paper towel lined plate to absorb the excess grease. Serve hot.

Tips

Another great seasoning to use is Creole. And with any fish fry, hot sauce is a must!

31 Creole Shrimp and Okra

Ready in 45 minutes

Serves 4 people

Calories: 404.5

Fat: 18

Net Carbs: 9

Protein: 51.25

Ingredients

- **2 pounds of raw jumbo shrimp, peeled/deveined**
- **1 yellow onion, julienned**
- **3 tablespoons of Creole seasoning**
- **4 tablespoons of bacon grease**

Kitchen Supplies

- ☐ Baking sheet with rim

- ☐ measuring spoons

Preparation

1. **Preheat oven to 350 degrees. Slice your onion into julienne slices and scatter evenly across the baking sheet. Cut your okra into bite sized pieces and scatter over the onions.**
2. **Next, lay your shrimp out evenly over top of the onions and okra.**
3. **Melt 4 tablespoons of bacon or use 4 tablespoons of olive oil to drizzle generously over the entire contents of the baking sheet.**
4. **Generously sprinkle Creole seasoning across everything; roughly 3 tablespoons**
5. **Place in the oven for 22-25 minutes or until shrimp is opaque and cooked thoroughly. Serve hot.**

Tips

Add bell peppers or a small amount of tomatoes to change it up a bit.

32 Blackened Flounder with Tomato Cream Sauce

Ready in 25 minutes

Serves 4 people

Calories: 455.75

Fat: 19.75

Net Carbs: 1

Protein: 62.25

Ingredients

- **8 flounder fillets**
- **¼ cup of heavy cream**
- **2 teaspoons of tomato paste**
- **1 teaspoon of blackening seasoning**
- **Salt and pepper (to taste)**
- **¼ cup of chicken broth**
- **½ cup of grated Parmesan**

Kitchen Supplies

- ☐ large baking dish

- ☐ medium sauce pan

- ☐ , whisk, measuring spoons/cups

Preparation

1. **Preheat oven to 325 degrees. Place your flounder fillets spaced evenly apart on the baking sheet and drizzle with olive oil then sprinkle salt and pepper to taste. Bake your fillets for 15-20 minutes or until they temp to 165 degrees.**
2. **In your sauce pan, add your chicken broth, heavy whipping cream, tomato paste, and blackening seasoning. Whisk the ingredients together over medium heat until fully incorporated. Then, add your Parmesan cheese and turn your heat down to low/medium. Whisk until fully incorporated and smooth.**
3. **Once your flounder is done, place two fillets, shingled, on a plate and drizzle your tomato cream sauce over top. Garnish with parsley for a nice touch.**

Tips
Saute some small shrimp in butter and garlic to put over top of your fillets for a restaurant style seafood entree.

33 Shrimp and Asparagus

Ready in 40 minutes

Serves 4 people

Calories: 474.5

Fat: 11.75

Net Carbs: 3.75

Protein: 51.25

Ingredients

- 2 pounds of raw jumbo shrimp, peeled and deveined
- 1 pound of asparagus, trimmed and chopped
- 2 tablespoons of olive oil
- 1 tablespoon of minced garlic
- 2 tablespoons of butter
- 6 ounces of Sauvignon Blanc
- Salt and pepper to taste
- 1 tablespoon of basil
- 4 tablespoons of grated Parmesan
- 1 tablespoon of parsley
- ½ cup of chicken broth

Kitchen Supplies

- ☐ Large saute pan

- ☐ cutting board and sharp knife

- ☐ Slotted spoon, whisk

Preparation

1. Heat olive oil in your large saute pan over medium heat. Add in your shrimp and your asparagus. Saute until the shrimp is cooked and no longer translucent. Set asparagus and shrimp aside.
2. Keep your heat set at medium and add the white wine to the empty saute pan. Cook until it reduces by half and add 2 tablespoons of butter,

minced garlic, salt and pepper, basil, and parsley. Whisk until smooth and fully incorporated.

3. Add your chicken broth and bring to a simmer then add back in your shrimp and asparagus. Simmer for 5-8 minutes. Sprinkle your Parmesan and toss it around. Remove from heat and serve immediately.

Tips

Add lemon juice for a lighter scampi style flavor or replace the seasonings listed with blackening seasoning for a kick.

34 Cajun Garlic Butter Shrimp

Ready in 1 hour

Serves 4 people

Calories: 515.75

Fat: 28.5

Net Carbs: 6

Protein: 51.75

Ingredients

- 2 pounds of raw jumbo shrimp, peeled/deveined
- 1 stick of butter
- 1 tablespoon of minced garlic
- 2 teaspoons of Cajun seasoning
- ¾ cup of Sauvignon Blanc
- 2 teaspoons of parsley
- ¼ cup of Parmesan
- 2 tablespoons of lemon juice

Kitchen Supplies

☐ large saute pan with lid

☐ whisk, measuring spoons, large spoon

Preparation

1. Place your lemon juice and white wine in your saute pan over medium heat. Allow it to simmer and reduce by half the amount of liquid.
2. Add in your stick of butter minus 1 tablespoon. Cut your stick of butter into small cubes to speed up the melting process. Turn your heat down to low/medium. Whisk frequently while the butter is melting to make sure that it doesn't break. Add in your minced garlic, parsley, and Cajun seasoning and stir well for 3-4 minutes. Pour your sauce in a bowl.
3. Next, turn your burn back to medium and add 1 tablespoon of butter. Once that melts, add your shrimp and cook until they are cooked thoroughly. Then add back in your sauce. Serve hot.

Tips
Dice up some peppers for a little more heat.

Beef, Pork, and Venison Recipes

35 Country Fried Steak

Ready in 1 hour

Serves 8 people

Calories: 388

Fat: 28

Net Carbs: 3

Protein: 28

Ingredients

- **(8) 3 ounce cubed steak pieces**
- **1/4 cup Bacon Grease**
- **1/2 teaspoon of dried dill weed**
- **1 egg**
- **1/2 teaspoon black pepper**
- **1 teaspoon of salt**
- **1 teaspoon paprika**
- **1 teaspoon thyme**
- **1 teaspoon garlic powder**
- **1 teaspoon rosemary**
- **1 teaspoon onion powder**
- **1 cup almond flour**
- **1 cup grated Parmesan cheese**
- **1/4 cup heavy whipping cream**

Kitchen Supplies:

☐ Large Deep Saute pan suitable for shallow frying

☐ Tongs or spatula for flipping

☐ 2 small mixing bowls

☐ Fork

☐ cutting board

☐ plastic wrap

☐ meat mallet

Preparation

1. Preheat a 1/4 cup of bacon grease in the saute pan. On a cutting board, lay each piece of cubed steak and cover with a piece of plastic wrap. Pound each piece with a meat mallet until flat. In one of the small mixing bowls, add dry spices, almond flour, and parmesan cheeses and blend well using a fork. In the other mixing bowl, add your egg and heavy cream and whip with your fork until well blended.

2. Place cubed steaks into the egg and cream mixture and coat each piece completely. Next, dip each piece of cubed steak into the Parmesan/almond flour coating and transfer directly to the pan.

3. Cook for 3-4 minutes on each side until each piece temps out above 155 degrees. Place on a paper towel lined plate to soak some of the grease up. Serve hot.

Tips

Other options than gravy, country fried steak also pairs well with Dijon style cream sauces, cheese sauces, as well as keto-friendly barbeque sauces.

36 Sauteed Veal in Lemon Pepper Cream Sauce

Ready in 30 minutes

Serves 4 people

Calories: 436

Fat: 26

Net Carbs: 2

Protein: 43.25

Ingredients

- **Eight 3 ounce cutlets of veal**
- **¼ cup of heavy whipping cream**
- **¼ cup of Parmesan**
- **¼ cup of chicken broth**
- **2 tablespoons of lemon juice**
- **1 teaspoon of garlic**
- **½ teaspoon of black pepper**
- **2 tablespoons of bacon grease**
- **Salt (to taste)**

Kitchen Supplies

- ☐ cutting board and a sharp knife

- ☐ large iron skillet

- ☐ small bowl

- ☐ whisk, measuring spoons/cups

Preparation

1. **In your large iron skillet, add 1 tablespoon of bacon grease over medium heat. Season your veal with salt to taste. Once your grease gets hot, add in 4 of your veal cutlets. You want them to sizzle when they hit the pan. Cook for 4 minutes on each side. This should give you an internal temperature of 165 degrees. If your veal is not seared enough at this point, raise the heat under your skillet to medium/high to further brown the outside without over**

cooking your veal. If you overcook your veal, it will be tough. Repeat the process starting with the second tablespoon of bacon grease. Once they are done, set your cutlets to the side and drain your drippings into a bowl to use for your sauce.

2. Do not clean your skillet in between; just make sure the majority of the drippings are out of the skillet. Then add your lemon juice and let it simmer over medium heat until the liquid reduces by half.

3. Add in your garlic, black pepper, salt to taste, and chicken broth. Still over medium heat, whisk until blended well and simmering again.

4. Add your heavy cream and whisk, then add in your Parmesan cheese. Continue to whisk until everything has been well combined. Turn your heat down to low/medium and stir frequently with your whisk to keep your sauce from breaking or scorching. Once the Parmesan has fully melted and the sauce is smooth, it is done.

5. Place 2 veal cutlets on a plate and drizzle with the lemon pepper sauce and serve.

Tips

Try using your favorite spices in the sauce instead of lemon juice and pepper. We love to change it up and add Italian seasoning.

37 Venison Roast

Ready in 6-7 hours

Serves 6 people

Calories: 349

Fat: 6.89

Net Carbs: 4.5

Protein: 62.75

Ingredients

- 3 pound venison roast
- ¼ cup of Worcestershire sauce
- 1 teaspoon of dried cilantro
- 1 teaspoon of garlic powder
- 1 teaspoon of onion powder
- ½ teaspoon of paprika
- ½ teaspoon of cumin
- 1 teaspoon of chili powder
- 1 cup of beef broth
- 4-6 cups of water
- 1 pound of radishes, trimmed with the root ends cut off, sliced in halves
- salt and pepper to taste

Kitchen Supplies

- ☐ cutting board and a sharp knife
- ☐ large crock pot
- ☐ medium mixing bowl
- ☐ Whisk, measuring spoons/cups

Preparation

1. In your medium mixing bowl, add your beef broth, dry seasonings, and Worcestershire sauce. Whisk to combine. Fill your mixing bowl with 3 cups of water and mix together to create a broth for your roast.

2. Place your roast in your crock pot and turn it on high. Pour your broth over the roast. Use up to 3 more cups of water in your crock pot to raise the liquid level to above the roast.
3. Let your roast cook for approximately 6 hours. You can begin to check it at 5 hours because depending on the style of crock pot, yours may cook a little faster. Your roast should be easy to tear apart with a fork. If it is still tough, set it for another hour.
4. Once your roast is fork tender, add in your radish halves and let them cook for another 30 minutes or so. You are looking for the radishes to be fork tender as well. Serve hot or portion out into 6 containers for a great meal prep.

Tips

Wanna add a little flare to it? Strain your roast and radishes and layer them in the bottom of a baking dish and top with bacon bits and cheddar cheese. Bake it in the oven until the cheese is melted and starting to blister.

38 Italian Meatballs

Ready in 30 minutes

Serves 4 servings

Calories: 274.25

Fat: 15.25

Net Carbs: .75

Protein: 32

Ingredients

- **1 pound of 80/20 ground beef**
- **1 tablespoon of Italian seasonings**
- **1 egg**
- **1 cup of grated Parmesan cheese**
- **1 tablespoon of bacon grease**

Kitchen Supplies

- ☐ large mixing bowl
- ☐ baking sheet with a rim
- ☐ measuring cups and spoons

Preparation

1. **Preheat the oven to 350 degrees. Melt your bacon grease and coat your baking sheet to prevent the meatballs from sticking before they produce their own grease.**
2. **In a large mixing bowl, combine all of the meatball ingredients and mix by hand until thoroughly incorporated.**
3. **Pinch off pieces of the meatball mix and roll around in the palm of your hand until you make a nice round ball. You want your meatballs to be about 1 inch in size. Place the meatballs in even rows on the coated baking sheet.**
4. **Cook the meatballs on the center rack in the oven for 15 minutes or until their internal temp is 165 degrees. Serve hot.**

Tips

These meatballs are great with low carb pizza sauce and mozzarella. They also make great appetizers.

39 Over-stuffed Pork Tenderloin

Ready in 2 hours, 15 minutes

Serves 6 people

Calories: 527.75

Fat: 36.75

Net Carbs: 3.75

Protein: 62

Ingredients

- **2 pound pork tenderloin**
- **1 pound of feta cheese crumbles**
- **1 yellow onion, julienne cut**
- **1 tablespoon of mince garlic**
- **4 tablespoons of bacon grease**
- **Salt and pepper (to taste)**
- **½ cup of shredded mozzarella**

Kitchen Supplies

- ☐ cutting board and a sharp fillet knife, sharp kitchen knife

- ☐ medium size mixing bowl

- ☐ medium saute pan with a lid

- ☐ large and deep baking pan

- ☐ plastic wrap and aluminum foil

- ☐ measuring spoons/cups/large spoon

- ☐ Food quality twine

Preparation

1. **Preheat oven to 300 degrees. Slice your onions on your cutting board with a sharp kitchen knife before beginning your tenderloin. Put 2 tablespoons of bacon grease in your saute pan and melt it over medium heat. As it is melting, add your onions to the grease. Cover and continue to cook for 5 minutes. Remove the lid and allow the onions to continue to cook until they are**

browned. Now add them to your mixing bowl along with your feta cheese, minced garlic, salt, and pepper. Combine your ingredients well and set aside.

2. While your onions are cooking, lay out your whole tenderloin long wise. This process is easy but don't rush it. From the cutting board up, roughly measure a ¼ inch and make a puncture with the tip of your fillet knife. Start with one end and work your way to the other making a "dotted line" down one side of your tenderloin. Now go back and with shallow strokes, cut down your "dotted line". Continue to cut deeper into your tenderloin a little bit more at a time keeping the thickness of the cut consistent. You want to fillet your tenderloin so that it rolls out into a ¼ thick sheet of pork.

3. Next, take the other two tablespoons of bacon grease and coat one side of your prepared pork and lay it face down. On the non coated side, lay an even layer of your onion and feta cheese stuffing.

4. This is where I like to get assistance to make it easier. Roll your sheet of pork up into a pinwheel, longwise. As you hold the tenderloin together, have someone else cut pieces of twine and tie them around the tenderloin, like you would tie up a sleeping bag, in 4 places to keep it from unrolling during the cooking process.

5. Place your stuffed tenderloin roll in your deep baking pan. Cover the pan with plastic wrap first, making sure to seal it around all 4 sides. Then cover the plastic wrap with aluminum foil. This will seal in the juices and keep it from drying out. Cook for 1 and a half to 2 hours depending on the thickness of your pork tenderloin. ¼ inch thickness will be done in 1 and a half hours. Check for an internal temperature of 165 degrees.

6. Pull your pork loin out of the oven and remove the aluminum foil and plastic wrap. Be careful. The steam will be really hot. Take the twine off the tenderloin and top with the rest of the stuffing. Over top of the stuffing, spread your mozzarella cheese evenly to keep the top stuffing in place.

7. Turn your oven to low broil or 450 degrees. Place the uncovered tenderloin on the top rack of your oven and cook for 5 minutes or until the cheese starts to blister on top. Remove it from the oven and let it stand for 10 minutes before serving.

Tips

Pork tenderloins are tricky the first few times your fillet the loin. If you don't want to pinwheel your tenderloin, cut it into pork chops and bake them the same way as above for 1 hour. Top them and broil to melt the cheese.

40 Bacon Wrapped Meatloaf

Ready in 1 hour, 15 minutes

Serves 10 people

Calories: 736.5

Fat: 61.8

Net Carbs: 1.6

Protein: 37.5

Ingredients

- 3 pounds of ground beef (80/20 is preferred)
- 1 pound of raw bacon
- 2 eggs
- 2 teaspoons of keto-friendly hickory barbeque seasoning
- ½ cup of keto-friendly barbeque sauce or ketchup
- ¼ cup of green bell peppers, diced
- ¼ cup of yellow onions, diced
- ½ cup of shredded cheddar cheese
- Salt and pepper (to taste)

Kitchen Supplies

- ☐ large mixing bowl
- ☐ large, loaf pan
- ☐ measuring spoons/cups

Preparation

1. Preheat oven to 350 degrees. In your loaf pan, place your bacon strips hanging half over the side of the dish on both sides evenly down the length of the pan. If you have enough bacon, you can wrap the ends too. You want two pieces of bacon to meet end to end in the center of the pan and line the side with enough hanging over the side to wrap over the top of your meatloaf.

2. In your large mixing bowl, combine your ground beef, eggs, cheddar cheese, bell peppers, onions, barbeque seasoning, salt, and pepper. Combine with your hands like kneading dough until the mixture is fully incorporated. Move the mixture over to your loaf pan and shape it with your hands. Wrap the

bacon slices over the top of the meatloaf and place it in the oven on the center rack. Bake for 45 minutes or until the middle of the meatloaf temps to at least 155 degrees (medium).

3. Once your meatloaf reaches the minimum internal temperature, turn your oven on low broil or 450 and cook for another 5-8 minutes until the bacon over top has become crispy.

4. Top with your choice of keto-friendly ketchup or barbeque sauce and serve.

Tips

Add some jalapenos or other spicy peppers for an extra kick. Serve with fresh guacamole, salsa, and sour cream as a toppings for a southwest flavor.

41 Restaurant Style Gorgonzola Steak

Ready in 40 minutes

Serves 4 people

Calories: 855

Fat: 52.25

Net Carbs: 10.75

Protein: 69.25

Ingredients

- **36 ounces of filet mignon beef**
- **1 cup of heavy whipping cream**
- **3 ounces of sun-dried tomatoes, julienne or diced**
- **8 ounces of Gorgonzola cheese crumbles**
- **½ cup of shredded Parmesan cheese**
- **1 teaspoon of minced garlic**
- **1 tablespoon of butter**
- **4 ounces of balsamic vinegar**
- **2 tablespoons of keto-friendly glycerin sweetener**
- **8 ounces of frozen spinach, thawed**
- **½ cup of chicken broth**

Kitchen Supplies

- ☐ medium sauce pan, small sauce pan

- ☐ grill or flat top for stove, tongs

- ☐ 2 whisks, measuring cups and spoons

Preparation

1. **Start your grill and set it to a medium heat/flame. You want it somewhere between 350 and 375 degrees. If you are using a flat top, wait until after you get your sauce started to heat it. Defrost your spinach and use a strainer to drain the water off. Set your spinach aside. Cut your sun-dried tomatoes to your preferred size if they are not already the size you want.**

2. Cut your filet beef into 3 ounce portions. You should have 12 total. (3 medallions for each person)
3. In your small sauce pan, simmer your balsamic vinegar for 10-15 minutes or until the reduction is half of the original amount. It will start to have a thin syrup-y texture but not quite enough to coat a spoon. Remove the pan from the heat and let cool for 5-10 minutes. Once the balsamic reduction reaches room temperature, add in your glycerin sweetener and whisk until the sauce is completely blended. Set aside to use for your drizzle over top of your dish.
4. In your medium sauce pan, melt your tablespoon of butter over low heat making sure not to allow it to get hot enough to 'break'. Use a whisk to keep the butter emulsified. Once your butterhas melted completely, add in your cup of heavy whipping cream and whisk the two together. Next add your chicken broth and whisk together.
5. Add in your minced garlic and 4 ounces of Gorgonzola cheese to your heavy cream/butter sauce and stir with a whisk frequently until it is smooth then add in your shredded Parmesan cheese and whisk until melted smooth. Adding both cheeses at one time tends to create clumping.
6. Once your sauce is near completion, place your filet medallions on the grill and cook to your favorite internal temperature.
7. Meanwhile, add your spinach and sun-dried tomatoes to your Gorgonzola sauce and continue to stir for 5 minutes. Next, add in your spinach and stir for another 5 minutes over low heat.
8. Place your filet medallions on your plate, shingled one on the other. Pour the Gorgonzola sauce evenly over the medallions. Next, drizzle a half tablespoon of your balsamic glaze over the middle of the dish and top with the remaining 4 ounces of Gorgonzola cheese as a garnish.

Tips

This dish is a little on the carby side but considering the alternative, 10.75 carbs is fantastic. With 19.25 grams of carbs in the entire dish coming from the balsamic glaze alone, you could back off the glaze to lower your carbs. This goes great over spaghetti squash or with a side of broccoli or asparagus. This dish makes for a great special occasion dinner or a "win someone over to keto" meal.

42 Shepherd's Pie

Ready in 1 hour

Serves 6 people

Calories: 418.25

Fat: 34.5

Net Carbs: 6

Protein: 13

Ingredients

- **1 pound of ground beef (preferably 80/20)**
- **1 bag of frozen green beans (any cut, I use Italian or french cut)**
- **½ pound of radishes, trimmed and root tips cut off, diced**
- **2 tablespoons of Worcestershire sauce**
- **1 tablespoon of keto-friendly steakhouse seasoning**
- **Salt and pepper (to taste)**
- **2 bags of frozen cauliflower rice**
- **2 tablespoons of heavy whipping cream**
- **2 ounces of cream cheese, softened**
- **4 tablespoons of butter**
- **½ teaspoon of garlic powder**
- **½ teaspoon of onion powder**
- **2 tablespoons of fresh chives**

Kitchen Supplies

- ☐ cutting board and sharp knife
- ☐ large saute pan with lid
- ☐ medium microwave bowl with lid
- ☐ hand mixer
- ☐ large baking pan
- ☐ slotted spoon, measuring cups and spoons

Preparation

1. Preheat oven to 350 degrees. Place your ground beef in the large saute pan and cover. Brown your ground beef making sure to crumble the meat into smaller pieces. Drain your ground beef but do not rinse it.
2. Microwave your frozen cauliflower rice as directed on the packages. Cook them for a minute longer than the maximum amount of time listed. Drain as much water off of your rice as possible using a cheesecloth or strainer.
3. Place hot cauliflower rice back in your mixing bowl. If the cauliflower has cooled down, place it back in the microwave with the lid on for another minute or two. It needs to be hot enough to melt butter. Add in your softened cream cheese, butter, garlic powder, heavy whipping cream, onion powder, and salt and pepper. Use your hand mixer to blend your cauliflower to a smooth texture much like mashed potatoes.
4. Meanwhile, trim the root ends off of your radishes. Cut your radishes into 4-6 pieces each. This should give you pieces that are roughly a half inch in size.
5. Add your steakhouse seasoning and Worcestershire sauce to your ground beef. Once you have stirred those in, add your radishes and frozen green beans. Cover the pan and heat until the radishes start to lose their red color and are fork tender. Remove the pan from the heat.
6. Next, place your ground beef/green beans/radishes in the bottom of your baking dish and spread out evenly. Then over top, spread or pipe your cauliflower mashed potatoes.
7. Bake in the oven for 20 minutes or until the top starts to brown and the edges are bubbly. Right before serving, garnish with fresh chives.

Tips

Add bacon bits to the ground beef or even use them as a garnish. Cheddar cheese is always a hit when I melt it over top.

43 Hamburger Steaks with Gravy

Ready in 40 minutes

Serves 6 people

Calories: 189.5

Fat: 11.5

Net Carbs: 2

Protein: 27.25

Ingredients

- 1 ½ pounds of ground beef, preferably 80/20
- 1 egg
- ¼ cup of grated Parmesan cheese
- ½ teaspoon of onion powder
- ½ teaspoon of salt
- ½ teaspoon of paprika
- ½ teaspoon of white pepper
- ½ teaspoon of xantham gum
- ¼ cup of beef broth
- 1 tablespoon of Worcestershire sauce

Kitchen Supplies

- ☐ flat surface to patty out burgers

- ☐ flat spatula, measuring cups and spoons

- ☐ large cast iron skillet

- ☐ large mixing bowl

Preparation

1. Preheat your skillet to medium heat.
2. In your large mixing bowl, combine your ground beef, egg, Parmesan cheese, onion powder, salt, paprika, and white pepper. Knead like dough with your hands until fully incorporated.
3. Separate the ground beef into 6 even amounts. Roll each amount around in your hand until you make a tight ball. Press down on a flat surface to patty the burger out.

4. Place the burgers in the hot skillet and let cook for 4-5 minutes on each side until the internal temperature is 165 degrees.
5. Remove the hamburger steaks and set them aside. Leave the juices in the skillet.
6. Reduce the heat under your skillet to low/medium and add in the Worcestershire sauce and the beef broth. Bring this to a simmer and stir occasionally to keep from clumping. As the beef broth reduces by about ½, you will see your gravy start to look like gravy, but a thinner consistency. Add your xantham gum a pinch at a time, stirring in between adding more. Give it a minute or two before you add another pinch. Xantham gum is a really good thickening agent. Also take into consideration that as it sits and cools it will thicken as well. Using too much xantham gum can cause your gravy to be clumpy and really thick.
7. Once your gravy is to the consistency that you want it, add back in your hamburger steaks. Cover the pan and let them simmer over low/medium heat for 5 minutes, flipping once during that time. Serve hot.

Tips

Add mushrooms to your gravy for a richer flavor.

44 Tennessee Whiskey Tips

Ready in 30 minutes

Serves 6 people

Calories: 570.25

Fat: 25.75

Net Carbs: .25

Protein: 57.25

Ingredients

- 3 pounds of filet mignon beef
- 2 teaspoons of minced garlic
- 375ml of Tennessee Whiskey (half of a standard bottle)
- Salt and pepper to taste
- 1 ½ cups of shredded pepperjack cheese

Kitchen Supplies

- ☐ cutting board and sharp knife

- ☐ grill, tongs

- ☐ large bowl with a lid

- ☐ oven safe small single serving dishes

Preparation

1. The night before you want to prepare this, cut your filet beef into 2 inch tips.
2. In a large bowl, add your Whiskey and your garlic and stir them together. Add your beef tips and cover. Marinade over night for best results.
3. When you are ready to prepare them, start your grill and get it to medium heat.
4. Turn your oven on low broil or 450 degrees.
5. Place your tips on the grill and cook until you have just below the actual internal temperature that you desire of your finished meal. (For example, if you want medium well tips, only grill your tips to medium.)
6. Spread tips evenly through 6 oven safe single serving bowls and top each with a ¼ cup of pepperjack cheese. Place the bowls in the oven on the

center rack and cook on low broil or 450 degrees only until the top cheese starts to blister. This shouldn't take more than 4 or 5 minutes. Serve hot.

Tips

Add caramelized onions before you top with cheese for richer flavor.

44 Tennessee Whiskey Tips

Ready in 30 minutes

Serves 6 people

Calories: 570.25

Fat: 25.75

Net Carbs: .25

Protein: 57.25

Ingredients

- **3 pounds of filet mignon beef**
- **2 teaspoons of minced garlic**
- **375ml of Tennessee Whiskey (half of a standard bottle)**
- **Salt and pepper to taste**
- **1 ½ cups of shredded pepperjack cheese**

Kitchen Supplies

- ☐ cutting board and sharp knife
- ☐ grill, tongs
- ☐ large bowl with a lid
- ☐ oven safe small single serving dishes

Preparation

1. The night before you want to prepare this, cut your filet beef into 2 inch tips.
2. In a large bowl, add your Whiskey and your garlic and stir them together. Add your beef tips and cover. Marinade over night for best results.
3. When you are ready to prepare them, start your grill and get it to medium heat.
4. Turn your oven on low broil or 450 degrees.
5. Place your tips on the grill and cook until you have just below the actual internal temperature that you desire of your finished meal. (For example, if you want medium well tips, only grill your tips to medium.)
6. Spread tips evenly through 6 oven safe single serving bowls and top each with a ¼ cup of pepperjack cheese. Place the bowls in the oven on the

center rack and cook on low broil or 450 degrees only until the top cheese starts to blister. This shouldn't take more than 4 or 5 minutes. Serve hot.

Tips

Add caramelized onions before you top with cheese for richer flavor.

45 Stuffed Bell Peppers

Ready in 45 minutes

Serves 4 people

Calories: 623.5

Fat: 55.4

Net Carbs: 6

Protein: 25.5

Ingredients

- **4 medium size red bell peppers**
- **1 tablespoon of balsamic vinegar**
- **1 tablespoon of olive oil**
- **4 ounces of cream cheese, softened**
- **1 teaspoon of basil**
- **1 teaspoon of minced garlic**
- **¼ cup of grated Parmesan**
- **Salt and pepper (to taste)**
- **Blue cheese crumbles**

Kitchen Supplies

- ☐ cutting board and a sharp knife
- ☐ medium size mixing bowl
- ☐ baking sheet
- ☐ large saute pan
- ☐ Rubber spatula
- ☐ measuring spoons/cups

Preparation

1. **Preheat oven to 350 degrees. On a cutting board, cut the top stem off each of your red bell peppers essentially making them into bowls. Remove all seeds and rinse.**
2. **In your large saute pan over medium heat, brown your ground beef, drain and rinse.**

3. Add your cream cheese to your ground beef and stir occasionally until it is fully melted into your ground beef and spread out evenly. Next, add your Parmesan cheese, basil, garlic, salt, and pepper and combine.
4. Take each bell pepper and coat the outside of it with a thin coat of olive oil. One tablespoon should be enough for all 4 but feel free to use more if necessary. Adding fats never hurt! Place each pepper standing up on the baking sheet.
5. Stuff each pepper with your ground beef mixture to roughly 2/3 – ¾ full. You need to leave about a ¼ inch at the top of each pepper.
6. Cover the baking sheet with aluminum foil and place in the oven for 10 minutes on the center rack.
7. Remove the aluminum foil and add 1 ounce of blue cheese crumbles on the top of each pepper then drizzle with balsamic vinegar. Serve hot!

Tips

Stuffed peppers are an easy and versatile keto meal. With this recipe, you can change the peppers to any color you want, change your spices and cheeses, and even change the filling to chicken instead.

46 Cajun Pork Chops

Ready in 30 minutes

Serves 6 people

Calories: 603.5

Fat: 39.5

Net Carbs: .5

Protein: 55.75

Ingredients

- **6 pork chops (you can use butterflied, bone in, or tenderloin cutlets, Just make sure to adjust your time for thicker or bone in chops)**
- **2 tablespoons of butter**
- **2 tablespoons of heavy whipping cream**
- **2 tablespoons of sour cream**
- **½ cup of grated Parmesan cheese**
- **1 tablespoon of Cajun seasoning**

Kitchen Supplies

- ☐ medium sauce pan

- ☐ baking sheet or saute pan (for frying or baking your pork chops)

- ☐ whisk, measuring spoons/cups

Preparation

1. **Preheat oven to 350 degrees if you are baking your pork chops. If you are frying them, place your pork chops in your saute pan and turn heat to medium. Season your pork chops with salt and pepper to your taste. Cook your pork chops until they reach an internal temperature of 165 degrees.**
2. **Meanwhile, in your medium sauce pan, melt your butter over low heat whisking frequently so that the butter doesn't break. Once the butter has melted, add your Cajun seasoning, heavy cream, and sour cream. Whisk your sauce until it is completely blended. Add your grated Parmesan cheese and continue to whisk until the sauce is hot and smooth.**
3. **Place your pork chops on a plate and smother them with your Cajun cream sauce.**

Tips

This pairs great with keto biscuits or corn bread for sopping up the left over sauce once you devour your pork chop!

Breakfast and Brunch Recipes

47 Faux-tater Hashbrown Casserole

Ready in 1 hour

Serves 8 people

Calories: 306.38

Fat: 24.7

Net Carbs: 8

Protein: 10.89

Ingredients

- **2 Small Spaghetti Squash (between the 2, it should yield 8 cups of cooked spaghetti squash. You can measure before you add it into the casserole)**
- **2 tablespoons Bacon Grease**
- **10 pieces of bacon**
- **½ cup Full Fat sour cream**
- **1 cup Chicken Broth**
- **½ cup Heavy Whipping Cream**
- **1 cup of shredded cheddar cheese / ½ cup shredded cheddar cheese**
- **½ tsp Paprika**
- **1 tbsp Onion powder (you can substitute a yellow onion if you want the texture but add 2 carbs per portion because they are higher in carbs)**
- **1 tsp Garlic powder**
- **Salt and pepper to taste**
- **2 oz full fat cream cheese**

Kitchen Supplies

- ☐ Baking dish (I use a 9x13 glass)
- ☐ measuring spoons/cups
- ☐ cutting board and sharp heavy duty knife

Preparation

1. **Preheat oven to 350 degrees. On a cutting board cut both spaghetti squash in half and scoop out the middle, much like a pumpkin.**

2. Line a baking sheet with aluminum foil. Use a basting brush to spread bacon grease inside and along the edges of the spaghetti squash.
3. Lightly salt and pepper the insides of each. You do not need to coat the outside. Place spaghetti squash on the foil lined pan upside down. Cook in the oven for approx. one hour or until you can squeeze the spaghetti squash and it seems soft.
4. Take out of the oven and lay to the side.

Tips

For a different texture, try grating radishes. Also, you can add other ingredients such as chicken, spinach, or bell peppers to add your own flare.

48 Turkey Spinach Egg Muffins

Ready in 25 minutes

Serves 12 individual muffins

Calories: 127

Fat: 8.5

Net Carbs: 1

Protein: 10

Ingredients

- 4 ounces of sliced deli meat turkey, diced
- ½ cup of sharp shredded cheddar
- 3 cups of fresh baby spinach
- salt and pepper to taste
- 1 teaspoon of onion powdered
- 12 eggs
- 2 tablespoons of heavy whipping cream
- 2 tablespoons of butter, melted

Kitchen Supplies

- ☐ 12 count muffin tin
- ☐ basting brush
- ☐ medium mixing bowl and whisk

Preparation

1. Preheat your oven to 350 degrees. Meanwhile, dice your deli turkey and also shred or chop your baby spinach.
2. Take your melted butter and coat each muffin cup with your basting brush to keep the muffins from sticking.
3. In your mixing bowl, add eggs, heavy whipping cream, salt, pepper, and onion powder. Whisk until thoroughly blended. Add the shredded cheddar cheese, spinach, and turkey to the eggs and fold all the ingredients together.
4. Evenly spread the mixture between each muffin cup. Each cup should be ¾ of the way full or lower as these tend to rise.

5. Bake the egg muffins for 15-18 minutes or until they start to turn golden brown. Serve hot.

Tips

Top with a fresh pat of sweet cream butter or add other ingredients to the muffins such as bacon, mushrooms, sun-dried tomatoes, or onions.

49 Old Fashioned Sausage Balls

Ready in 25 minutes

Serves 30 pieces

Calories: 89.5

Fat: 6.75

Net Carbs: .5

Protein: 5.25

Ingredients

- 1 cup of almond flour
- 1 pound of spicy breakfast sausage in a roll
- 1 cup of shredded cheddar cheese
- 1 teaspoon of salt
- 1 teaspoon of paprika
- 1 egg
- 1 teaspoon of water

Kitchen Supplies

- ☐ large mixing bowl
- ☐ 2 baking sheets, parchment paper
- ☐ measuring cups/spoons

Preparation

1. Preheat oven to 325 degrees. In your mixing bowl, add all of your ingredients and combine thoroughly with your hands like kneading dough.
2. Place parchment paper over both baking sheets.
3. Next, Roll the dough into 1 inch balls and place evenly across both pans.
4. Cook for 15 minutes or until the sausage balls temp to 165 degrees. Serve hot or cold.

Tips

Dip these in french onion dip or queso for a great appetizer idea and dip in sugar free pancake syrup for breakfast and brunch,

Sides and Sauces

50 Loaded Radishes

Ready in 40 minutes

Serves 6 people

Calories: 180

Fat: 14.5

Net Carbs: 2.5

Protein: 8

Ingredients

- **1 pound of radishes, trimmed with the root tips cut off**
- **Salt**
- **½ cup shredded cheddar cheese**
- **2 tablespoons of dried chives**
- **¼ cup of bacon bits**
- **6 tablespoons of sour cream**
- **4 tablespoons of butter**
- **6-8 cups of water**

Kitchen Supplies

- ☐ Large pot
- ☐ cutting board and sharp knife
- ☐ baking sheet with a rim
- ☐ slotted spoon, measuring cups and spoons

Preparation

1. **Preheat oven to 350 degrees. Start your 6-8 cups of water in a large pot to boil. As you trim the radishes, add them to the pot. Bring the radishes to a rolling boil. About 10 minutes in, check for fork tenderness. Remove the pot from the heat and drain your radishes.**
2. **On your baking sheet, line your radishes up leaving a little room in between. Now go back and smash each of them with a fork keeping them individual. Melt the butter and drizzle it over top of all the radishes being generous as you go.**
3. **Next, top your radishes with bacon bits and cheddar cheese.**

4. Place the radishes in the oven to bake for 10 minutes or until cheese is melted and starts to blister.
5. Right before you serve them, top each one with a dollop of sour cream and chives.

Tips

Get creative and change up your toppings. Since radishes taste similar to potatoes, they are easily paired with most any meal.

51 Ranch Dressing (Dry Mix)

Ready in 10 minutes

Yields 1/2 pint

3 tablespoons equals 1 store package

Calories: 12

Fat: 0

Net Carbs: 1

Protein: .5

Ingredients

- **2 teaspoons salt**
- **4 tablespoons parsley**
- **3 teaspoons dill weed**
- **2 teaspoons dried chives**
- **4 teaspoons garlic powder**
- **4 teaspoons onion powder**
- **2 teaspoons black pepper**
- **2 teaspoons basil**

Kitchen Supplies

- ☐ bowl
- ☐ spoon

Preparation

1. **Combine all ingredients in a bowl and mix well. Place in an air tight mason jar for storage.**

Tips

Add 3 tablespoons to the following for a wet dressing.
> 1/2 cup sour cream
> 1/2 cup mayonnaise
> 2 tablespoons heavy cream

52 Garlic Roasted Radishes

Ready in 1 hour, 15 minutes

Serves 4 people

Calories: 148.5

Fat: 12.5

Net Carbs: 2.75

Protein: 1.5

Ingredients

- **1 pound of radishes, trimmed at the ends.**
- **2 teaspoons of Italian seasoning**
- **5 tablespoons of butter**
- **1 teaspoon of minced garlic**
- **Salt (to taste)**
- **6 cups of water**

Kitchen Supplies

- ☐ cutting board and a sharp knife
- ☐ large baking sheet with rim
- ☐ large pot
- ☐ measuring spoons/cups

Preparation

1. **Preheat oven to 350 degrees. Start your 6 cups of water to boil. As you trim your radishes you can add them to the large pot. Boil your radishes until just before fork tender. Drain your radishes and spread them out across your baking sheet.**
2. **Melt your butter in the microwave. Add your minced garlic and salt to the butter and stir well. Drizzle your garlic butter over your radishes and toss to completely saturate them.**
3. **Bake your radishes in the oven for 20 minutes or until they start to brown and fork tender. Serve hot.**

Tips
If you want to add a crispier outside, at the end, broil your radishes for 3-5 minutes until you achieve the texture you want.

53 Fried Green Tomatoes

Ready in 30 minutes

Serves 6 people

Calories: 279.75

Fat: 25.25

Net Carbs: 4.5

Protein: 5

Ingredients

- **3 green tomatoes (home grown is the best)**
- **¾ cup of almond flour**
- **¾ cup of grated Parmesan cheese**
- **4 tablespoons of bacon grease**
- **Salt and pepper to taste**
- **½ teaspoon of onion powder**
- **½ teaspoon of garlic powder**
- **½ teaspoon of paprika**
- **½ teaspoon of cumin**
- **½ teaspoon of oregano**
- **½ teaspoon of rosemary**
- **½ teaspoon of thyme**
- **1 egg**
- **¼ cup of heavy whipping cream**

Kitchen Supplies

- ☐ 2 small mixing bowls
- ☐ a large plate and paper towels
- ☐ fork, tongs
- ☐ cutting board and a sharp knife
- ☐ large saute pan

Preparation

1. Place your 4 tablespoons of bacon grease in the large saute pan and begin to melt it over low/medium heat.
2. Slice your tomatoes no more than ¼ of an inch thick.
3. In one of your small mixing bowls, combine the heavy cream and egg. Beat with a fork until fully blended. This will be your egg wash.
4. In the other small mixing bowl, combine the rest of your dry ingredients and mix well. This will be your "breading".
5. Check the bacon grease to be sure it has reached a temperature of at least 350 degrees. If you need to turn the heat up, make sure the temp is above 350 before you add your tomatoes but not above 400.
6. Take your tomato slices one at a time and coat them in the egg wash then dredge them through the "breading" to coat each side.
7. Place each slice in the bacon grease and let cook on each side until golden brown. As with most anything breaded, do not turn or flip more than you have to or the breading will fall off before you get it out of the grease.
8. Place your fried green tomatoes on a paper towel lined plate to soak up any excess grease.

Tips

These make fantastic "how to entice your family to get on board" bait especially for those who have had the original ones from Juliet, GA.

54 Roasted Brussel Sprouts

Ready in 35 minutes

Serves 4 people

Calories: 121

Fat: 10.25

Net Carbs: 2.5

Protein: 1.5

Ingredients

- **1 pound of fresh brussel sprouts**
- **4 tablespoons of butter**
- **½ teaspoon of minced garlic**
- **½ teaspoon of paprika**
- **½ teaspoon of rosemary**
- **½ teaspoon of thyme**
- **½ teaspoon of oregano**
- **Salt and pepper to taste**

Kitchen Supplies

- ☐ cutting board and a sharp knife
- ☐ small mixing bowl
- ☐ baking sheet with rim
- ☐ measuring spoons, spoon

Preparation

1. **Preheat oven to 350 degrees. Trim the stems off of your brussel sprouts and slice them in halves. Evenly spread them across your baking sheet.**
2. **In your mixing bowl, microwave your butter to melt it. Add in your minced garlic, rosemary, thyme, paprika, salt, and pepper and mix.**
3. **Pour your butter sauce over your brussel sprouts making sure to coat all of them evenly.**
4. **Bake in the oven for 25-30 minutes. Serve hot.**

Tips

Change up your seasonings with an Italian blend or use a keto-friendly steakhouse seasoning.

55 Grilled Asparagus

Ready in 20 minutes

Serves 4 people

Calories: 80

Fat: 6

Net Carbs: 2.5

Protein: 3

Ingredients

- **1 pound fresh asparagus**
- **2 tablespoons Bacon Grease**
- **8 cups water to boil**
- **2 tablespoons salt**
- **8 cups ice water**
- **Black pepper to taste**

Kitchen Supplies

- ☐ cutting board and sharp knife
- ☐ 2 large stock pots
- ☐ Grill

Preparation

1. Begin with preheating your grill to 350 degrees.
2. Meanwhile, bring 8 cups of water to a rapid boil, set up your second stock pot with ice water, and melt your bacon grease in the microwave.
3. Wash and trim the stalky ends off the asparagus. The ends are a purplish white and tend to be stringy and tough.
4. Drop asparagus into the boiling water and let cook for 3-4 minutes until tender, blanching the asparagus.
5. Remove from boiling water with tongs and transfer asparagus immediately to the stock pot with ice water to stop the cooking process quickly.
6. Once the asparagus is cool, remove from the ice water and dry with a paper towel.
7. Toss asparagus in melted bacon grease and place on the grill.

8. Heat on the grill for 3-4 minutes until you start to see grill marks, then remove, sprinkle with black pepper, and serve

56 Green Bean Almondine

Ready in 30 minutes

Serves 4 people

Calories: 239.5

Fat: 21.4

Net Carbs: 4

Protein: 8

Ingredients

- 1 pound of fresh green beans
- ½ cup of slivered almonds
- 3 tablespoons of bacon grease
- 6 pieces of bacon, crumbled
- 1 teaspoon of garlic powder
- 1 teaspoon of onion powder
- Salt and pepper (to taste)

Kitchen Supplies

- ☐ tongs or slotted spoon
- ☐ large iron skillet
- ☐ measuring spoons/cups

Preparation

1. Preheat your bacon grease in your skillet. Once melted, toss in your almonds. Saute your almonds over medium heat for 5-10 minutes depending on how crunchy you prefer them. Add in your garlic powder, onion powder, salt and pepper and combine.
2. Next, add in your green beans and crumbled bacon. Toss them around until fully coated and cover. Let your green beans cook for 20 minutes or until your preferred texture.
3. Remove from heat and serve.

Tips
Add a diced Serrano or crushed red pepper flakes for some heat. Replace the bacon with diced pancetta and top with Parmesan for an Italian flare.

57 Honey Mustard

Ready in 5 minutes

Serves 4 servings

Calories: 400

Fat: 48

Net Carbs: 0

Protein: 0

Ingredients

- ¼ cup of mustard
- ¼ cup of mayonnaise
- 1 tablespoon of keto friendly glycerite style sweetener

Kitchen Supplies

- ☐ small bowl and a whisk

Preparation

1. Place all ingredients in a bowl and whisk until smooth.

58 Mexican Cauli-rice

Ready in 15 minutes

Serves 4 people

Calories: 95.25

Fat: 0

Net Carbs: 3

Protein: .8

Ingredients

- **1 bag of frozen cauliflower rice**
- **2 tablespoons of chicken broth**
- **1 tablespoon of tomato paste**
- **1 teaspoon of Tajin seasoning**
- **1 diced roma tomato**
- **Salt (to taste)**

Kitchen Supplies

- ☐ cutting board and a sharp knife
- ☐ medium saute pan
- ☐ slotted spoon, measuring spoons

Preparation

1. **Microwave your frozen cauliflower rice as directed on the package.**
2. **Remove the cauliflower rice from the microwave and pour it into your saute pan with your chicken broth, tomato paste, seasoning, and salt. Mix completely and bring to a simmer. Add a tablespoon more of chicken broth should it seem dry.**
3. **Once your cauliflower rice is done, toss in your diced roma tomatoes and serve immediately.**

Tips
Add some jalapenos or other spicy peppers for an extra kick.

59 Grandpa's Georgia Gold Barbeque Sauce

Ready in 5 minutes

Serves 10 servings

Calories: 9.25

Fat: 0

Net Carbs: 2

Protein: 0

Ingredients

- ¾ cup of reduced sugar ketchup
- 1/3 cup of yellow mustard
- 2 tablespoons of Worcestershire sauce
- 1 tablespoon of lemon juice

Kitchen Supplies

- ☐ a mason jar

Preparation

1. Place all ingredients in the mason jar and put the lid on it. Shake the jar until the ingredients are mixed well.

Tips

Add a little sugar free glycerite sweetener for a hint of honey flavor.

60 Sauteed Spinach

Ready in 20 minutes

Serves 4 people

Calories: 67.75

Fat: 7

Net Carbs: 1

Protein: .5

Ingredients

- **2 pounds of fresh baby spinach**
- **1 teaspoon of minced garlic**
- **2 tablespoons of olive oil**
- **1 tablespoon of lemon juice**
- **Salt and pepper to taste.**

Kitchen Supplies

- ☐ large saute pan

- ☐ Large spoon, measuring spoons

Preparation

1. **In your saute pan, add the minced garlic and olive oil. Heat over low/medium heat. Once your oil is hot, add your spinach and stir to coat it all.**

2. **Next, add your salt, pepper, and lemon juice. Once the spinach is partially wilted, it is done.**

Tips

Add bacon bits with the olive oil and add walnuts at the end.

61 Cauliflower "Faux" Tater Salad

Ready in 1 hour

Serves 8 people

Calories: 185.75

Fat: 17.5

Net Carbs: 3.75

Protein: 2.25

Ingredients

- **1 large head of cauliflower, trimmed into small florets**
- **¼ cup of yellow onion, diced**
- **1 cup of celery, diced**
- **10 strips of bacon, crumbled**
- **½ cup of mayonnaise**
- **Salt and pepper to taste**
- **1/8 cup of mustard**
- **1 teaspoon of dill weed**
- **ice water**

Kitchen Supplies

- ☐ Large Mixing bowl
- ☐ cutting board and sharp knife
- ☐ Spatula, measuring spoons and cups
- ☐ Steamer pan

Preparations

1. **Clean and cut your cauliflower into small florets and place in the steaming pan. Cook for 5 minutes until al dente. Next, take the cauliflower and submerge it in cold ice water to stop the cooking process.**
2. **Dice your onions and celery and place aside.**
3. **Combine your mayonnaise, mustard, dill weed, salt, pepper, bacon, onion, and celery completely.**
4. **Drain the cauliflower and dry with paper towels or cheese cloth.**

5. Combine cauliflower with mayonnaise and mustard mixture with a spatula. Serve cold.

Tips

Try blending in some cheddar cheese or feta for a unique twist.

62 Fat Bomb Salad

Ready in 5 minutes

Serves 1 person

Calories: 674

Fat: 61

Net Carbs: 4

Protein: 30

Ingredients

- **1 cup fresh baby spinach**
- **2 tablespoons bacon bits**
- **2 tablespoons blue cheese crumbles**
- **1 diced boiled egg**
- **2 tablespoons keto friendly Caesar dressing**
- **2 tablespoons chopped pecans**

Kitchen supplies

- ☐ Salad bowl

- ☐ Salad tongs

Preparation

1. **Combine all ingredients in a salad bowl and toss until full incorporated. Serve in a chilled bowl.**

Tips

Try adding balsamic vinegar instead of Caesar dressing and replace the pecans with crushed walnuts.

63 Deviled Eggs

Ready in 40 minutes

Serves 12-24 people

Calories (each half): 52

Fat: 4.5

Net Carbs: .5

Protein: 3

Ingredients

- **12 Large eggs**
- **1/4 cup mayonnaise**
- **1/4 cup mustard**
- **1 teaspoon baking soda**
- **1 teaspoon sugar free relish**
- **6 cups water**
- **a sprinkle of paprika**

Kitchen supplies

- ☐ Small mixing bowl
- ☐ Large pot
- ☐ Hand mixer
- ☐ small spatula
- ☐ Zippered Sandwich bag and scissors

Preparation

1. **Add a teaspoon of baking soda and 6 cups of water to a large pot over high heat. As the water starts to come to a rolling boil, set a timer for 10 minutes.**
2. **In a small mixing bowl, add your mayonnaise, mustard, and relish then blend well.**
3. **Once the eggs have finished boiling, drain the hot water and replace with cold. Add ice cubes to speed up the process. After the eggs are chilled, peel the shells off and cut the eggs in half.**

4. Scoop the egg yolks into the mixing bowl with the mayonnaise and mustard mixture and mix with a hand mixer on medium until smooth.
5. With your spatula, scoop all the filling into a zippered sandwich bag and remove as much air as possible. Cut one of the bottom corners of the bag with scissors to make a piping bag.
6. Pipe your filling into the egg white halves and place on a plate. Garnish with a sprinkle of paprika.

Tips

You can get really creative with deviled eggs. Try changing up your ingredients such as replacing your mustard with hot sauce and topping with crumbled blue cheese for a buffalo style egg.

64 Pesto Cauliflower Risotto

Ready in 20 minutes

Serves 4 people

Calories: 277

Fat: 21

Net Carbs:7

Protein: 10

Ingredients

- **1 medium head of cauliflower, riced or 1 frozen bag of cauliflower rice**
- **8 tablespoons Basil Pesto**
- **1/2 cup grated Parmesan**
- **1 ounce sun-dried tomatoes diced small**
- **1/4 cup Chicken Broth**
- **1/4 cup Heavy Whipping Cream**
- **1 teaspoon salt**

Kitchen supplies

- ☐ One medium saute pan
- ☐ Large spoon
- ☐ measuring cups

Preparation

1. **First, prepare your cauliflower rice. You can either cut it and put it in the food processor to create "rice" or you can buy prericed cauliflower from your store. Whether frozen or fresh, cook in microwave until soft, and has an al dente texture.**
2. **Meanwhile, preheat your saute pan with chicken broth added to it over low/medium heat. After 2-3 minutes, add cooked cauliflower rice and soak completely with chicken broth.**
3. **Next, add your heavy cream, Parmesan cheese and sun-dried tomatoes and mix thoroughly.**
4. **Lastly, turn the heat off and add pesto and blend well. Serve hot.**

Tips

Try changing up the sun-dried tomatoes and pesto and add with 1/2 cup of dry Marsala wine before the chicken broth and let it reduce. Then add ingredients from that point. Also add in mushrooms with the cauliflower rice for a great Marsala risotto.

65 Cauli-Mac and Cheese

Ready in 40 minutes

Serves 6 people

Calories: 227

Fat: 15.25

Net Carbs: 4

Protein: 8.25

Ingredients

- **2 bags of frozen cauliflower florets**
- **¼ cup of chicken broth**
- **1 cup of shredded sharp cheddar cheese**
- **½ cup of heavy whipping cream**
- **1 teaspoon of rotisserie chicken seasoning**
- **1 ounce of pork rinds crushed**
- **2 tablespoons of butter**
- **pinch of xantham gum**
- **1 teaspoon of ground mustard**
- **salt (to taste)**

Kitchen Supplies

- ☐ 2 small mixing bowls

- ☐ baking dish (I use glass)

- ☐ medium sauce pan, whisk

- ☐ large spoon, measuring cups, and spoons

Preparation

1. **Preheat your oven to 350 degrees.**
2. **Microwave your cauliflower as directed on the packages and then spread them out in your baking dish.**
3. **In your sauce pan, add your heavy whipping cream, chicken broth, cheddar cheese, and rotisserie seasoning, ground mustard, and whisk over low/medium heat until smooth. Add xantham gum a pinch at a time**

until you get to the consistency you want. Pour your cheese sauce over your cauliflower and toss to coat evenly.

4. In one small mixing bowl, crush your pork rinds to bread crumb consistency and melt your butter in the microwave using the other small bowl. Combine the two and coat the pork rinds with the butter. Layer the top with the butter/pork rind mixture.

5. Bake in the oven for 20 minutes or until the top of the dish is golden brown and the edges are bubbly.

Tips

Add bacon or for a spicier version, add buffalo chicken and top with crumbled blue cheese.

66 Southern Fried Cabbage

Ready in 30 minutes

Serves 6 person

Calories: 188.5

Fat: 12

Net Carbs: 8.75

Protein: 7.75

Ingredients

- **1 large head of cabbage, shredded or chopped**
- **10 strips of bacon**
- **3 tablespoons of bacon grease**
- **4 ounces of vidalia onion, diced**
- **Salt and pepper to taste**

Kitchen supplies

- ☐ Large saute pan with lid
- ☐ Large bowl
- ☐ tongs or spatula
- ☐ cutting board and sharp knife

Preparation

1. **Put the 3 tablespoons of bacon grease in the saute pan and turn on low heat to start melting it.**
2. **Either shred or cut your cabbage to how you prefer it and put it aside in your large bowl**
3. **Cut your vidalia onion into small diced pieces and add to the bacon grease in the saute pan. Turn the heat up to medium/high and cook until they start to brown.**
4. **Crumble your bacon into the saute pan with the onions. Next, begin to incorporate your cabbage into the saute pan stirring and coating all the cabbage in the bacon grease and onion mixture.**
5. **Cover your saute pan with a lid and let it cook for approximately 15 minutes stirring every 5 minutes. Serve hot.**

Tips

Add some crushed red pepper for a spicy kick or add in a ¼ cup of sugar free maple syrup for a sweet flavor. Get creative and add both!

67 Southern Fried Okra

Ready in 35 minutes

Serves 6 person

Calories: 312.75

Fat: 24.75

Net Carbs: 5.25

Protein: 13.5

Ingredients

- **1 pound of fresh okra, chopped**
- **½ cup of almond flour**
- **½ cup of coconut flour**
- **1 cup of Parmesan**
- **¼ cup of heavy whipping cream**
- **1 egg**
- **½ teaspoon of onion powder**
- **½ teaspoon of cayenne pepper**
- **½ teaspoon of cumin**
- **1 teaspoon of salt**
- **4 tablespoons of bacon grease**

Kitchen supplies

- ☐ Gallon sized zipper storage bag
- ☐ large saute pan
- ☐ spatula, fork, measuring cups and spoons
- ☐ medium mixing bowl
- ☐ cutting board and sharp knife
- ☐ Large plate and paper towels

Preparation

1. **Over low heat, add bacon grease to your saute pan so that it can be melting.**
2. **Next, chop your okra, removing the stems as you go. Set aside.**

3. In a medium mixing bowl, add your heavy cream and your egg and beat with a fork until well combined to create an egg wash.
4. Add your okra to the egg wash and mix until each piece is fully coated.
5. Turn your bacon grease up to medium heat. You want your frying grease to be at least 350 degrees.
6. In your zippered storage bag, combine coconut flour, almond flour, Parmesan cheese, cayenne, cumin, salt, and onion powder. Close the bag and shake until all the ingredients are mixed well.
7. Take your okra a few pieces at a time and toss into the dry mix in the bag. Keep adding okra until all the pieces are fully coated with "breading".
8. Add your okra a handful at a time to the hot bacon grease carefully and let them fry on each side for about 4 minutes each. You shouldn't have to flip them but once or twice. Be sure not to stir or flip them too much as the breading will fall off before it is cooked all the way.
9. Put your fully cooked okra on a large plate lined with a paper towel to absorb the excess grease before serving.

Tips

Try replacing the above seasonings with an Italian seasoning blend and top with low carb marinara sauce and mozzarella cheese for a great side option for Italian dishes.

68 Southern Creamed Spinach

Ready in 20 minutes

Serves 4 people

Calories: 208.75

Fat: 17

Net Carbs:5.25

Protein: 12

Ingredients

- **2 pounds of fresh baby spinach**
- **1 teaspoon of minced garlic**
- **1 teaspoon of salt**
- **1 teaspoon of black pepper**
- **½ cup of heavy whipping cream**
- **½ cup of shredded Parmesan cheese**
- **1 ounce of cream cheese**

Kitchen Supplies

- large saute pan with lid
- spatula or large spoon
- measuring cups and spoons

Preparation

1. **Place your large saute pan over low/medium heat. Add in your heavy whipping cream and cream cheese. Stirring occasionally, heat until smooth. Next, add in your Parmesan cheese, minced garlic, salt, and pepper. Stir continuously until sauce is smooth and to a similar thickness to Alfredo sauce.**
2. **Once the sauce is ready, add in your spinach and stir until completely saturated. Place the lid over the pan and let the spinach wilt. Stir occasionally if necessary. Wilting of the spinach should take no more than 5 minutes. Serve hot.**

Tips

Want to add a different flavor? Try replacing the garlic with my recipe for dry ranch seasoning.

69 Thanksgiving Gravy

Ready in 10 minutes

Serves 16 people

Calories: 233.5

Fat: 26

Net Carbs: .02

Protein: .01

Ingredients

- **2 cups of turkey drippings (chicken drippings work great too!)**
- **1 tablespoon heavy whipping cream**
- **1/2 teaspoon of xantham gum**

Kitchen supplies

- ☐ Small sauce pot

- ☐ whisk

Preparation

1. **Add your drippings to your sauce pot over low/medium heat.**
2. **Add your heavy whipping cream and whisk until blended.**
3. **Next, slowly sprinkle in xantham gum. You want to make sure you add it slowly, sprinkling evenly to prevent clumps. Whisk consistently until you start to see the gravy thicken.   Serve immediately.**

Tips

For a thicker gravy, add a little more xantham gum. You want to add it slowly as above starting with a pinch at a time because a little really does go a long way.

70 Dirty Cauli-rice

Ready in 40 minutes

Serves 6 people

Calories: 321

Fat: 27.5

Net Carbs: 4

Protein: 11.75

Ingredients

- **2 bags of frozen cauliflower rice**
- **2 tablespoons of bacon grease**
- **1 pound of ground beef (preferably 80/20)**
- **1 tablespoon of Cajun seasoning**
- **¼ cup of diced yellow onion**
- **¼ cup of diced green bell pepper**
- **1 tablespoon of crushed red pepper flakes**
- **salt (to taste)**

Kitchen Supplies

- ☐ cutting board and sharp knife
- ☐ large iron skillet with lid
- ☐ slotted spoon, measuring cups and spoons

Preparation

1. **In your large iron skillet, melt your bacon grease and add your diced yellow onions and bell peppers. Saute your onions and peppers for 3 minutes and then add your ground beef to the skillet. Brown your ground beef but do not drain it. Add in your Cajun seasoning and crushed red pepper flakes.**
2. **Microwave your bags of cauliflower rice as directed on the package. Add your cauliflower rice to the skillet and combine all ingredients. Add salt to taste and serve.**

Tips

Add diced jalapenos or Serrano instead of red pepper flakes for extra heat.

71 Egg Salad

Ready in 40 minutes

Serves 6 people

Calories: 351.75

Fat: 31.75

Net Carbs: 2.25

Protein: 17.25

Ingredients

- **One dozen large eggs**
- **½ cup of mayonnaise**
- **1/8 cup of mustard**
- **¼ teaspoon of paprika**
- **1 teaspoon of sugar free relish**
- **1 cup of celery, diced**
- **¼ cup of fresh chives, chopped**
- **¼ cup of diced yellow onion**
- **1 teaspoon of baking soda**
- **6 cups of water**

Kitchen supplies

☐ Large Pot

☐ Large mixing bowl

☐ Spatula, sharp knife, measuring spoons and cups

☐ cutting board

☐ hand mixer

Preparation

1. **In your large pot, add baking soda, water, and eggs with the shell on and set on high heat. As the eggs begin to hit a rolling boil, set a timer for 10 minutes. Once the eggs are done, drain the hot water and add cold water to the pot. Add ice cubes to aid in the cooling down process.**

Let the eggs stand until they are room temperature or colder. Peel each egg and slice them in half. Set the eggs aside for later.

2. In your large mixing bowl, add your mayonnaise, mustard, paprika and relish. Next, scoop your egg yolks into the bowl with the mayonnaise and mustard blend. Use your hand mixer on low setting and whip the ingredients until smooth.

3. Next, toss in your onion, crumbled bacon, chives, and celery. Mix well.

4. Take your boiled egg whites and cut them up in larger chunks adding them to your mixture in the bowl. Take a rubber spatula and fold the egg whites into the mayonnaise and mustard blend without damaging them too much. Serve cold.

Tips

Try replacing the mayonnaise and mustard with my honey mustard recipe and add a tablespoon of crushed red pepper!

72 Rosemary Brussel Sprout Casserole

Ready in 30 minutes

Serves 4 people

Calories: 306.38

Fat: 24.7

Net Carbs: 8

Protein: 10.89

Ingredients

- (2) 11 ounce bags of frozen brussel sprouts in the steam-in bags. (you may use fresh also but you have to pre cook them before you begin this recipe. Frozen does not affect the quality of this recipe and it takes a substantial amount of time off the preparation.)
- 3 tbsp of bacon grease or butter
- 4 ounces of bacon bits
- 3/4 cup of shredded sharp cheddar cheese
- 1/2 cup of shredded Parmesan cheese
- 1 tsp of dried crushed red pepper flakes
- 2 tsp of rosemary
- 1 tsp of garlic powder
- 1 tsp of onion powder
- 1/2 cup of heavy whipping cream
- 1 egg

Kitchen supplies

- ☐ 9x9 baking pan

- ☐ large mixing bowl, medium mixing bowl, and mixing spoon

- ☐ cutting board and sharp knife

- ☐ Measuring cups and spoons

- ☐ Whisk

Preparation

1. Preheat oven to 350 degrees. Melt bacon grease or butter in the microwave for 30 seconds to a minute until it is completely melted. Pour bacon grease in the bottom of your baking pan to prevent from sticking as well as flavoring the recipe.
2. Take the brussel sprout bags and place them both on a microwave safe plate in the microwave for 3 minutes on high. You do not want to cook them, you only want them to defrost slightly so you can cut through them without them falling apart. On a cutting board, take a sharp knife and trim any remaining stems left, then cut the brussel sprouts in halves and add to your large mixing bowl and set aside.
3. In the medium mixing bowl, add your egg, and heavy cream. Whisk until fully combined and then add your dry seasonings and bacon bits and mix thoroughly. Then add your shredded cheeses and fold into the sauce.
4. Take the finished mixture and pour into the large mixing bowl over top of the brussel sprouts and coat well. Pour all of this into the baking pan and smooth flat. Cook for 20 minutes or until the sides start to bubble and the cheese starts to turn golden brown. Serve hot.

Tips

Add more cheese and bacon bits over top for a more polished product.

73 Cauliflower Fritters

Ready in 30 minutes

Serves 10 people

Calories: 173.5

Fat: 13.5

Net Carbs: 4

Protein: 6.75

Ingredients

- **1 large head of cauliflower, riced**
- **1 egg**
- **1 cup of almond flower**
- **¾ cup of shredded cheddar cheese**
- **1 teaspoon of onion powder**
- **1 teaspoon of garlic powder**
- **Salt and Pepper to taste**
- **4 tablespoons of bacon grease**

Kitchen Supplies

- ☐ cutting board and sharp knife

- ☐ large saute pan

- ☐ food processor

- ☐ 1 large microwave safe mixing bowl with lid

- ☐ large plate, paper towels

- ☐ rubber spatula or spoon, flat spatula, measuring cups and spoons

Preparation

1. **Cut your cauliflower into small florets and add them a little at a time to a food processor until the entire head has been riced.**
2. **Place the riced cauliflower in a large microwave safe bowl and gently lay the lid on top, not securing it. Place the bowl in the microwave for 10 minutes. Let stand with the lid off for 5 minutes then drain the water off your cauliflower rice in a cloth or strainer.**

3. In the large saute pan, melt your bacon grease over low/medium heat until the temperature reaches 350 degrees.
4. Next, add your egg, almond flour, cheddar cheese, garlic powder, onion powder, salt, and pepper in with the cauliflower rice. Combine well.
5. Make patties the size of the palm of your hand and add them to your hot grease. Cook over medium heat for 4 minutes on each side or until golden brown and reach an internal temperature of 165 degrees.
6. Lay your cauliflower fritters on a paper towel lined plate to absorb the excess grease. Serve hot.

Tips

This is a great meal prep dish for those busy days where cooking is the least of your concerns.

74 Skillet "Faux" Taters

Ready in 30 minutes

Serves 6 person

Calories: 74.5

Fat: 7

Net Carbs:2.5

Protein: .75

Ingredients

- **1 pound of radishes trimmed, the root tips cut off, and sliced thin**
- **3 tablespoons of bacon grease**
- **½ cup of diced yellow onion**

Kitchen supplies

- ☐ large saute pan
- ☐ slotted spoon, measuring cups and spoons
- ☐ cutting board and sharp knife

Preparation

1. **Over medium heat, melt your bacon grease in a large saute pan.**
2. **Dice your yellow onion into the size pieces you prefer. I prefer small diced as they brown a lot faster.**
3. **Put the onions in the saute pan with the bacon grease and cook until golden brown.**
4. **Add in your sliced radishes and cook for 15 minutes or until they are fork tender and the red skin turns a pale pink to white. Serve hot.**

Tips

Bacon crumbles make a great addition to this recipe!

75 Keto "Cornbread" Dressing

Ready in 30 minutes

Serves 6 people

Calories: 546

Fat: 56

Net Carbs: 4.5

Protein: 10.25

Ingredients

- 1 cup almond flour
- 1/4 cup flax seed meal
- 1/2 cup coconut flour
- 1 raw egg, 1 boiled egg
- 3 tablespoons bacon grease
- 1 cup chicken or turkey drippings (You can use chicken broth but drippings are so much tastier and loaded with fat!)
- 2 ounces of shredded chicken meat or turkey meat
- 1 teaspoon salt
- 1/2 teaspoon baking powder
- 1/4 cup heavy whipping cream
- 1/4 yellow onion, diced

Kitchen supplies

- ☐ 8x8 baking pan
- ☐ spoon for mixing
- ☐ medium mixing bowl

Preparation

1. Preheat oven to 325 degrees and coat the bottom of your baking pan with bacon grease. If you do not have a preboiled egg on hand, now would be the time to prepare it.
2. In your mixing bowl, combine almond flour, flax seed meal, coconut flour, diced onion, 1 raw egg, heavy whipping cream, baking powder, 3 bacon grease, and salt. Stir until mixed into a dough texture.

3. Add dough mixture to the baking pan and spread out evenly. Cover pan with aluminum foil and bake for 15 to 20 minutes. You are looking for a crumbly texture but no burned edges.
4. Remove from the oven and let dressing cool slightly. Crumble the dressing throughout the pan and then add chicken or turkey meat, chipped up boiled egg and chicken or turkey drippings and stir around until all ingredients are wet but not mushy. You want just slightly damp.
5. Recover pan with aluminum foil and bake for 10 minutes. Serve hot.

Tips

When boiling your eggs, add a teaspoon of baking soda to your water. When you remove them from the heat, drain the hot water from the pot and add ice water. 10 minutes later you should be able to peel your eggs without a problem. If you like your dressing more 'wet', add more drippings or broth.

76 Parmesan Sauteed Asparagus

Ready in 20 minutes

Serves 4 people

Calories: 99

Fat: 7.5

Net Carbs: 2.5

Protein: 5

Ingredients

- **1 lb of fresh asparagus**
- **2 tbs of bacon grease or butter**
- **1 tsp of minced garlic**
- **1 tbs of grated Parmesan**
- **2 tbs of bacon bits**
- **Salt and Pepper to taste**

Kitchen supplies

- ☐ Large Saute Pan with lid

- ☐ Utensil for stirring

- ☐ cutting board and a sharp knife

- ☐ measuring spoons

Preparation

1. In a saute pan over medium heat, add 2 tablespoons of bacon grease or butter until melted.
2. Rinse your asparagus and cut off any purple or white stalk ends. The ends tend to have a bitter stringy texture so trimming is necessary for this recipe. Dice the remaining stalks of asparagus into quarters and add to the saute pan.
3. Next, add the minced garlic, bacon bits, salt and pepper.
4. Cover your saute pan with the lid. Saute over medium heat, stirring occasionally, for approximately 10 minutes or until the asparagus starts to sear a golden brown.

5. **Remove your pan from the heat and sprinkle Parmesan over top. Replace the lid and let your asparagus sit for 2 to 3 minutes to allow for the Parmesan to start to melt. Serve hot.**

Tips

As another option, melt blue cheese crumbles over top in place of the Parmesan.

77 Broccoli Salad

Ready in 20 minutes

Serves 8 people

Calories: 309.5

Fat: 30.75

Net Carbs: 3.5

Protein: 7.5

Ingredients

- **1 head of fresh broccoli**
- **10 slices of bacon, crumbled**
- **¼ cup of diced red onion**
- **½ cup of shredded mild cheddar cheese**
- **1 cup of mayonnaise**
- **1/8 cup of powdered erythritol**
- **2 tablespoons of white vinegar**

Kitchen supplies

- ☐ Large mixing bowl

- ☐ Utensil for stirring

- ☐ cutting board and a sharp knife

- ☐ measuring spoons

- ☐ small mixing bowl, whisk

Preparation

1. **Cut your broccoli into small size florets and add to your mixing bowl.**
2. **Next, dice your red onion and crumble your bacon. Add these and the cheddar cheese to your mixing bowl. Combine ingredients until it is mixed well.**
3. **In a small mixing bowl, add your mayonnaise, powdered erythritol, and white vinegar and whisk thoroughly.**
4. **Pour the sauce over your broccoli salad mix and combine well evenly coating all of the broccoli.**

5. Either store for later or chill and serve cold.

Tips

Add some diced jalapenos or Serrano peppers for a little kick. Just be sure to take the seeds out before you add them to your broccoli salad.

78 Peppered Sausage Gravy

Ready in 20 minutes

Serves 4 people

Calories: 585

Fat: 53.5

Net Carbs: 5.25

Protein: 17.5

Ingredients

- **1 pound of hot sausage**
- **8 ounces of cream cheese**
- **1 tsp of black pepper**
- **½ cup of heavy whipping cream**
- **½ tsp of salt**
- **¼ cup of water**

Kitchen supplies

- ☐ Large saute pan with lid

- ☐ rubber or plastic whisk

Preparation

1. **In your large saute pan, crumble the sausage with your hands. Set heat to medium and stir occasionally until completely brown. Do NOT drain!**
2. **Dice your cream cheese up into 1 inch cubes and place in the pan with the sausage. Turn your heat down to low/medium and stir frequently.**
3. **Once your cream cheese has almost completely melted, add your black pepper and heavy cream. Stir with a whisk until the sauce around the sausage is smooth.**
4. **Add a ¼ cup of water if the sauce is too thick. You can adjust this up or down according to the consistency that you prefer.**
5. **Pour over keto friendly biscuits and serve! (See my biscuit recipe in this book)**

Tips

If you accidentally put too much water in the sauce, simply add xantham gum a pinch at a time until you get your preferred consistency back.

79 Broccoli Cauli-rice Casserole

Ready in 30 minutes

Serves 6 people

Calories: 161.5

Fat: 20.2

Net Carbs: 4.7

Protein: 8.3

Ingredients

- **1 bag of frozen broccoli**
- **1 bag of frozen cauliflower rice**
- **1/2 cup of chicken broth**
- **1 cup of shredded sharp cheese**
- **1/2 cup sour cream**
- **1/2 teaspoon garlic powder**
- **1/2 teaspoon black pepper**
- **1 teaspoon of salt**
- **1 ounce of crushed pork rinds**
- **1 tablespoon of butter melted**
- **2 tablespoons bacon grease for coating your baking pan**

Kitchen Supplies

- ☐ Small sauce pan
- ☐ measuring cups
- ☐ whisk
- ☐ fork
- ☐ small bowl

Preparation

1. Preheat oven to 350 degrees. Coat your baking dish with either bacon grease or butter to keep the dish from sticking.
2. Meanwhile, microwave your broccoli as the package directs and rough cut it into bite sized pieces. Next, microwave the cauliflower rice according to the package. Set both to the side for now.

3. To make the sauce, add ½ cup of chicken broth, 1 cup of sharp cheddar cheese, ½ cup of sour cream, garlic powder, salt and pepper to your sauce pan. Stir continuously with a whisk over low to medium heat as it combines and the cheese melts into a creamy sauce.
4. In a glass baking pan, add the cooked cauliflower rice and broccoli. Pour your cheese sauce evenly over top.
5. In a separate bowl, crush one ounce of pork rinds until they are the consistency of bread crumbs. Microwave your tablespoon of butter then combine it with the pork rinds until they are all fully coated. Top your casserole with the pork rind mixture then bake for 20 minutes.

Tips

This recipe is so versatile. You can add bacon, chives, or even bacon, sausage or chicken to complete a one dish meal.

80 Fully Dressed Guacamole

Ready in 30 minutes

Serves 4 people

Calories: 174.6

Fat: 14.75

Net Carbs: 4

Protein: 2.5

Ingredients

- **2 small avocados, ripe**
- **2 drops of orange extract**
- **¼ cup rough chopped cilantro**
- **1 roma tomato, diced small**
- **1/2 of a Serrano pepper, diced small**
- **1 tablespoon of lime juice**
- **1 tablespoon of finely chopped red onion**
- **1 teaspoon of minced garlic**
- **½ teaspoon of salt**

Kitchen Supplies

- ☐ small mixing bowl
- ☐ measuring cups
- ☐ cutting board and sharp kitchen knife
- ☐ fork
- ☐ table spoon

Preparation

1. **Dice and chop all of your produce first. Then slice each avocado down the middle, length-wise, all the way around. Twist the two pieces apart and remove the seed with your knife or table spoon.**
2. **Scoop out the meat of the avocado into a mixing bowl and mash with a fork until as chunky or as smooth as you want it.**
3. **Add Lemon extract, lime juice, and salt. Mix well.**
4. **Add your diced produce next and blend until well incorporated.**

Tips

Serve with cheese chips, celery, or sliced raw peppers for dipping. You can also add salsa, sour cream, cheese and some jalapenos on top to make a 5 layer dip.

81 Giblet Gravy

Ready in 15 minutes

Serves 10 people

Calories: 15.25

Fat: 1.25

Net Carbs: .05

Protein: .25

Ingredients

- **1 bag of giblets**
- **1 cup of chicken broth**
- **1 teaspoon of heavy whipping cream**
- **½ teaspoon of xantham gum (maybe a pinch more if needed)**
- **1 tablespoon of butter**
- **Salt and pepper to taste**

Kitchen Supplies

- ☐ medium sauce pan

- ☐ whisk

- ☐ measuring cups/spoons

Preparation

1. **In a medium sized sauce pan over medium heat, whisk to combine your giblets, butter, chicken broth, heavy whipping cream, salt, and pepper. Bring the contents to a boil then reduce heat to low/medium. Add in your xantham gum a pinch at a time until your gravy will coat a spoon. Remove from heat and serve immediately.**

Tips

Use your drippings from your bird instead of chicken broth for a richer flavor.

82 Roasted Cauliflower

Ready in 30 minutes

Serves 6 people

Calories: 41.25

Fat: 5

Net Carbs: 4.5

Protein: 2.75

Ingredients

- **1 large head of cauliflower, trimmed and cut into florets**
- **2 tablespoons of melted bacon grease**
- **1 teaspoon of garlic powdered**
- **salt and pepper to taste**
- **2 teaspoons of crushed red pepper flakes**
- **1 teaspoon of oregano**

Kitchen Supplies

- ☐ cutting board and sharp knife
- ☐ baking sheet with a rim
- ☐ slotted spoon, measuring cups and spoons, basting brush
- ☐ small bowl

Preparation

1. **Preheat oven to 375 degrees. Trim and cut your cauliflower into florets and space them out on the baking sheet.**
2. **Melt 2 tablespoons of butter in a small bowl. Add in the onion powder, garlic powder, and oregano. Use a basting brush to coat each piece of cauliflower then sprinkle crushed red pepper flakes over all of the cauliflower.**
3. **Bake in the oven for 15 minutes or until the cauliflower starts to brown on the edges. Serve hot.**

Tips

Try using Italian seasoning and topping with Parmesan seasoning right at the end.

83 Zucchini and Squash Casserole

Ready in 1 hour

Serves 6 people

Calories: 240

Fat: 16

Net Carbs: 5.25

Protein: 12.9

Ingredients

- 3 medium zucchini
- 3 medium to large yellow squash
- ½ cup of heavy whipping cream
- 1 egg
- ¾ cup of shredded cheddar cheese
- ¾ cup of shredded Gruyere cheese
- ¼ cup of bacon bits
- Salt and pepper (to taste)
- 1 teaspoon of onion powder

Kitchen Supplies

- ☐ cutting board and a sharp knife
- ☐ medium size mixing bowl
- ☐ 9x9 baking dish
- ☐ Rubber spatula
- ☐ fork, measuring spoons/cups

Preparation

1. Preheat oven to 350 degrees. On a cutting board, slice your your zucchini and squash into 1/8 to ¼ of an inch in thickness. If you want your squash to have a crunch to it, cut them ¼ inch thick. The thinner they are cut, the softer they will get as they cook.
2. Layer your zucchini and squash in the pan evenly spreading them out.
3. In your mixing bowl, add your heavy cream and egg. Beat with a fork until the two are combined. Add in your onion powder, salt, pepper, ½ cup of your

cheddar cheese and ½ cup of Gruyere cheese and mix well. Pour the mixture over top of your squash and zucchini evenly. Top the casserole with the other ¼ cups of each cheese and sprinkle your bacon bits on top for a garnish.

4. Bake in the oven for 40 minutes or until the cheese is blistering on top and the sides are bubbly.

Tips

Add a protein to make this recipe a one dish meal.

84 Cheddar Cheese Sauce

Ready in 20 minutes

Serves 6-8 people

Calories: 148.5

Fat: 13.5

Net Carbs: 2

Protein: 5.5

Ingredients

- 1 cup of shredded cheddar cheese
- ¾ cup of chicken broth
- ½ cup of heavy whipping cream
- ½ teaspoon of ground mustard
- Salt and pepper to taste
- ½ teaspoon of paprika
- 1 teaspoon of garlic powder
- 1 teaspoon of onion powder

Kitchen supplies

- ☐ Medium sauce pan
- ☐ whisk or spatula

Preparation

1. Add all of your ingredients to your sauce pan and set to low/medium heat. Stir frequently until smooth. Serve hot.

Tips

You can add this sauce to so many entrees. Also, try adding keto friendly ingredients like mushrooms, broccoli, bacon, or chives. This also makes a great cheese sauce for dipping keto pretzels and breads in.

COMING SOON:
FAT-TASTIC ENDULGENCES
KETO-FIED DESSERTS
October 2018

DEEP FRIED AND KETO-FIED
VOLUME 2
January 2019

CPSIA information can be obtained
at www.ICGtesting.com
Printed in the USA
BVHW01s0852200518
516773BV00003B/188/P